For my dad and my brother

who taught me that life is short and health is everything.

Don't wait.

Contents

Acknowledgments

Thanks to my mom who introduced me to the fitness industry when I was 16, starting me on a lifelong career in health and wellness. Thank you to my high school boyfriend and forever husband who is always there for me through the crazy ups and downs of life. Thanks to my sweet rescue pup and running partner who brings me daily joy. Thank you to all my clients, friends and family for their support.

Thank you to all my teachers over the years for sharing your wisdom and for expanding me in endless ways, especially: Beth Shaw, Susan Bianchi, Kendell Reichhart, Joshua Rosenthal and all the teachers at Integrative Institute of Nutrition (IIN). Thanks to FOODMATTERS TV who exposed me to the documentary films Food, Inc. and Hunger For Change, which started me on a quest to heal myself and help others do the same with yoga, self-care and food.

I am thankful for the support of my friends, especially my writing accountability coach Jill McCullough, fellow IIN health coach Page Wasti, writing inspiration Ian Wasti, CSA farmer Lisa Duff and reliable friend Gaby Fishpaw.

Thank you to my nephew Jake Kendrick for spending his day off to film yoga segments and take pictures with me. Thanks to my website designer and friend Monique Savits for being fast, fun and endlessly creative.

Thank you to Towson University professor JoAnne Broadwater and to the students in her News Editing class: Timothy Barbalace, Brian Baublitz Jr., Christina Billos, Deion Broxton, Rachel Buchanan, Lauren Ferguson, Jai-Leen James, Chanda Kumar, Julie Lasheski, Aaron Mazer, Jessica Oyawale, Monet Stevens, Jared M. Swain, Max Venezia, Brandon Wajbel. Your heartfelt participation in the editing process made this book possible. Having the opportunity to work with students who sat in the same classroom as me, 25 years later, was both nostalgic and rewarding.

Extra thanks to Chanda Kumar for designing the book cover and interior layout. Working with this talented, creative and passionate student was a joy.

Thank you Under Armour for providing me with the best athletic gear on the planet!

Finally, as hard as it is to be thankful for Lyme disease, Hashimoto's autoimmune thyroid disease and the injuries and pain that pushed me to my edge and brought me to my knees, the education I have acquired is priceless and for that I am grateful.

Special thanks to you, the reader, for stretching your mind and body.

Introduction

Flexibility is just as much mental as it is physical. It's how you respond when things don't go as planned, whether it's a race day or an average day. How do you react when circumstances change? Do you waste energy freaking out, internalizing your stress? Or do you shake it off, go with the flow, come up with a new plan or take a different path?

When I was diagnosed with Lyme disease and autoimmune thyroid disease, I wasted years of my life fighting fatigue, feeling sorry for myself and resisting slowing down. I dealt with the diagnosis by pushing through, surviving on coffee, sugar and painkillers instead of embracing the situation and giving myself the time and TLC to heal. As a result, my health got progressively worse.

Ironically, during those years, I was working in the health and fitness industry as an instructor at Canyon Ranch Resort Spa and later as the marketing director at The Maryland Athletic Club. I felt pressure to be energetic, fit and healthy, yet I was exhausted and sick. Little by little, I learned to accept my diagnoses and began to open my mind to new ways of thinking. I stopped teaching step aerobics and began taking yoga. I started to add in more self-care like acupuncture, chiropractic and massage.

The yoga experience was so profound, I soon took a YogaFit® teacher training and studied for two years to become a certified yoga teacher. I eventually quit my marketing job and began pursuing a full-time career in yoga. I continued to experiment with many healing modalities, self-care techniques and styles of stretching.

I founded Flexible Warrior in 2001 with the intention of bringing chillpower and flexibility to tight athletes. I was fortunate to teach yoga for a variety of athletes and teams like the University of Maryland Terrapins Men's basketball team and the Baltimore Ravens football team. I taught yoga classes for athletes and private sessions that attracted runners, triathletes, golfers and athletic students of all types.

Next, I filmed a series of Flexible Warrior DVDs produced by Spinervals. My coolest experience to date was helping Olympic athlete Suzanne Stettinius stay flexible and recovered while she trained for five sports leading up to the 2012 summer Olympics in London. I'll never forget the moment while I was stretching her in my basement yoga studio when she said, "When I make it to the Olympics I'm taking you with me." Cheering her on at the Olympic games was unreal.

Throughout all these fantastic experiences, I still struggled with my health. There were times I had flare-ups of pain and fatigue that were so intense I couldn't leave the house for days. As a fitness professional, I was embarrassed, so I kept it mostly a secret. Only my husband really knew how bad it was. The self-care and healing techniques I learned were helping, but there was still something missing.

After a particularly long and painful flare up in the winter of 2012, I hired holistic health coach Kendell Reichhart at Natural Vibrant Health. She and I immediately clicked. I had seen dozens of doctors over a fifteen year span who only offered me antidepressants and painkillers to mask my symptoms. My intuition was telling me there was another way.

Although I thought my diet was pretty healthy, Kendell looked at my nutrition and suggested some big changes. Within months I felt much better and a year later my symptoms had improved so dramatically that I decided to enroll in school with Integrative Institute of Nutrition (IIN)® to become a health coach myself.

As I continued on my healing journey, I realized that the self-care, yoga and stretching techniques I was doing were also helpful for athletic clients looking to recover faster and improve flexibility. The anti-inflammatory superfood diet I was adopting was beneficial for everyone because it can prevent and even heal many diseases and reduce the pain and stiffness caused by inflammation.

This book is not about burning fat, finding a magic diet or sculpting a flawless body. It's not about doing exactly the right stretches for your sport or eating a perfect diet. It's about balance, experimentation and the kind of flexibility that can open up your mind and body in ways you've never imagined. Flexibility is power and freedom in how you think, how you move and how you eat.

> *"May all beings everywhere be happy and free.*
>
> *And may the thoughts and actions of my own life contribute, in some way,*
>
> *to that happiness and to that freedom for all."*
>
> **- Ancient Sanskrit Mantra**

Approach This Book With Flexibility

The theme of this book is to inspire you to create more flexibility and chillpower in your life to balance out your strength and willpower. It's not intended to provide you with an exact to-do list. My goal is to expose you to a less-is-more approach and a wide variety of self-care, stretching and diet options, all of which I have personally experienced. We briefly address each topic as an overview, but it will be your job to delve deeper, research further and experiment on your own to see what works for you. There are many other techniques beyond what is listed in this book.

Over the 25 years I've been in the fitness industry, I have studied many different techniques and I've seen a lot of trends. It was Lyme and thyroid disease that expanded my education beyond traditional fitness and into self-care. My focus on flexibility and recovery was a necessary shift in order to sustain my career and my own health. In doing so, I'm now able to support others to be more flexible and healthy. My hope with this book is that you too will gain a few tips to help you become more resilient and balanced. Fitness is not just about sit-ups and sweat. It's also about nutrition, flexibility and recovery.

The field of nutrition and fitness is always evolving. Our bodies, chemistry and goals are each unique. One size never fits all. Approach this book with a flexible, open mind and a sense of curiosity. See what appeals to you and experiment with a few new self-care techniques, stretching styles or dietary theories. Ultimately, your goal is to create your own customized Flexible Warrior plan and to put together the tools and team of practitioners to help you get and stay more flexible, recovered and healthy.

Good luck! Stay in touch. I'd love to hear from you!

Karen Dubs
Facebook.com/flexiblewarrior
Twitter: @flexiblewarrior
Instagram: flexiblewarrior
Youtube.com/flexiblewarrioryoga

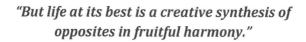

"But life at its best is a creative synthesis of opposites in fruitful harmony."

- Martin Luther King Jr.

PART I

Willpower & Chillpower

The balance of opposites includes extremes like hot and cold, hard and easy, win and lose and challenge and surrender. Sadly these days, the balance of opposites is more about pushing as hard and fast as possible to the point of collapse, finding stillness only to tune into some electronic device, or over indulging on unhealthy food and drinks, then jumping into the latest restricting fad diet.

While stop and go are opposites, I'll be encouraging you to find a less extreme sense of balance, where you can approach your self-care, stretching and eating with more flexibility and joy in order to experience less burnout and injury. To create more balance in your life, you'll need to put as much effort into your chillpower as you do your willpower.

FLEXIBLE WARRIOR - Willpower & Chillpower

The concept behind Flexible Warrior is the balance of the opposites: calm energy, stability with mobility, power and peace, willpower and chillpower.

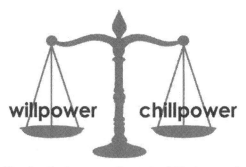

Willpower: The strength of purpose, self control and drive to carry out one's decisions despite obstacles. The determination, focus, courage, perseverance and strength of a warrior. A person with willpower won't take the easiest route, even though they know there will be less hardship. They choose the harder route because it's more rewarding.

Chillpower: The ability to let go and be at peace with what is. To consciously choose to relax and surrender into a state of calm in order to recharge and rebuild. To practice flexibility in mind and body. To go with the flow. To be resilient and pliable, capable of bending without breaking and able to respond to unplanned or altered circumstances and changing conditions.

Many of us have the strength and willpower to do hard things, but lack the chillpower required to rest and recharge. My goal is to help inflexible warrior types recover and be more resilient. My hope is that, like me, you will benefit from more self-care, stretching and anti-inflammatory superfoods.

People often call me "The Flexible Warrior" which always makes me laugh. Compared to my hard-core clients and friends, I'm more of a wimp than a warrior. Alongside my yoga friends, I'm closer to Tin Man than Gumby. No extreme races or crazy pretzel poses for me. I never really considered myself a warrior either. My job is to help keep the *real* warriors recovered and flexible. I realize now we are all a warrior at some level. Being fit and healthy is as much about resting, eating well and flexibility as it is about discipline and training hard.

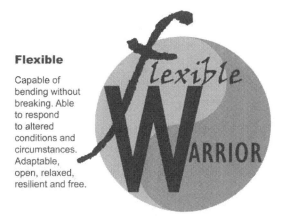

Flexible

Capable of bending without breaking. Able to respond to altered conditions and circumstances. Adaptable, open, relaxed, resilient and free.

Warrior

A brave fighter. Someone who is willing to endure and sacrifice for a higher purpose and engage in a challenge or battle, stepping out of his or her comfort zone for the greater good.

The Balance of Opposites

Warriors have great willpower, but when balanced with chillpower and flexibility, they are stronger and more resilient.

A warrior can be a gentle, loving, stay-at-home mom, a busy business executive, someone battling a disease, an athlete or a defender of our great nation. No matter your battle, if you have the determination to rise up, take action and fight for what you want, you are an empowered warrior. The other choice is to be a helpless victim who lets life happen or blames others for their circumstances. To be your best, knowing how to eat well and take care of yourself needs to be a priority. A commitment of just 10-30 minutes a day is all it takes. I think that's doable no matter how busy you are.

Our body has the amazing ability to heal when we listen to the messages it sends and take action. There are dozens of choices along our healing journey. Ultimately each of us has to follow our own intuition and find our own sense of balance between willpower and chillpower. The Flexible Warrior approach is about opening our mind and body to new healing paths. Instead of being mentally and physically rigid, we become more resilient and empowered by embracing flexibility and finding our own sense of balance.

Namaste

My soul honors your soul.

I honor the place in you where

the entire universe resides.

I honor the light, love, truth,

beauty & peace within you,

because it is also within me.

In sharing these things

we are united, are the same,

we are one.

- Author Unknown

"Winners never quit and quitters never win."

– Vince Lombardi

"Fall seven times and stand up eight."

– Japanese Proverb

"People usually fail when they are on the verge of success. So give as much care to the end as to the beginning; then there will be no failure."

– Lao-tzu

1

Willpower

More is More

This is not a pep talk. I have a feeling you already know a thing or two about willpower and how invigorating it is to do hard things and earn the rewards. You know that dedication, sacrifice, hard work, pushing to the edge of your comfort zone and avoiding temptation can bring a sense of joy. Once you've achieved your goal and look back, it's always worth it.

Who would disagree with the statement, "Where there's a will, there's a way?" All warriors have willpower. Warriors are willing to face challenges and persevere despite discomfort. People with willpower don't just talk, they do! Those who lack willpower do a lot of talking, but don't follow through. Willpower is the willingness to roll up our sleeves, do hard things, walk through the fire and take action.

In yoga, the word for action is "karma." We often think karma is good or bad, but in reality it is neutral and simply means that we get what we give. Based on our intentions and desires, we choose our actions and our actions have consequences. We must choose wisely, because what we do will eventually come back. Believing in karma gives me a sense of peace, because I don't have to worry about what others do. I know the universe will take care of it. All I need to do is focus on my own actions, have faith and be patient with the process.

"What you do speaks so loudly that I cannot hear what you say."

- Ralph Waldo Emerson

Exercise is addictive because it boosts endorphins, lifts our mood, keeps us feeling and looking youthful and increases energy and confidence. People get hooked on the runner's high and can't get enough. The interesting paradox is that for all its benefits, exercise can also lead to injury, especially when it's done to an extreme.

Anyone who has ever played a sport or trained hard with consistency has likely dealt with exercise-induced pain or injuries. Bad form is not always the culprit. Many injuries are caused by over-training and lack of quality rest. There is pain from the discomfort of pushing your edge and there is pain from injury. Don't confuse the two.

Injury and pain are often a side effect of too much willpower. The more-is-more mentality can lead to pushing over your edge through the overuse and misuse of many different kinds of training. This has led to many warrior-types training too hard or too frequently. They end up injured and broken down instead of stronger and faster. The more-is-more approach can backfire unless it is balanced with chillpower.

If you have a more-is-more mentality, try experimenting

"You can go hard. You can go long. But you can't do both. The popularity of high-intensity interval training (HIIT) has many people misusing it. If you're doing more than 2-3 HIIT workouts a week, you're either going to get an overtraining injury or you aren't doing HIIT."

- Award-winning Fitness Professional Jonathan Ross

with committing some of your workout time to easy, flexibility-based recovery workouts. Doing so may help you feel more balanced and less fatigued. Investing part of your training time in self-massage, stretching or meditation can often benefit you more than 10 extra minutes of cardio or strength training.

I believe that you get what you give and results come to the warriors who are willing to dig deep and step outside of their comfort zone. I also feel it's equally important to create balance in our training and lives and embrace our chillpower.

Never Give Up

To achieve success in life, we must be willing to practice with commitment for a long period of time. When we decide we want something and commit to reaching our goal, we don't ever want to give up. We believe if we give up, we fail. However, as head coach John Harbaugh said during the Ravens 2014 season, "There is no success without failure."

The Sanskrit word for "never give up" is Abhyasa. It's all about commitment, consistent practice and overcoming obstacles that are there to test our will and faith. Abhyasa is the willingness and determination to get back up after you've been knocked down and to try again.

I remember when I first learned about Abhyasa and its opposite Vairagya (always let go). I was in my early 30s and was at a yoga teacher training. I was in a "never give up" phase of my life where I was constantly challenging myself and working toward being successful, healthy and fit.

Even though I was studying yoga, my approach and pace was fast and aggressive. I wanted it all and I wanted it now. At the time, I didn't have much balance in my life. I was all about "more-is-more" and "never give up." Even after being diagnosed with Lyme and Hashimoto's autoimmune thyroid disease, I never stopped for one minute to surrender. Slowing down never crossed my busy mind.

My reward was that I had accomplished a lot and had a career I loved. I was the marketing director for the best health club in Baltimore and was teaching Yoga and Spinning™ for the Baltimore Ravens football team. It was an exciting time in my life. I even trained for my first 5K that year, while I was on antibiotics for Lyme. I traveled constantly for yoga trainings, worked my marketing job and taught fitness classes. I was having issues with my health, but I didn't want to give anything up. One day, my knees literally buckled while I was teaching a step aerobics class. I taught the rest of that class sitting on the stage and I knew that something had to change. I took myself off the fitness schedule that day. I started taking yoga the next week. When I surrendered, my healing journey was able to begin.

A few weeks after that incident, I learned about Abhyasa and Vairagya. I got chills as the teacher described the two wings of a bird and how we need both wings to fly. We need discipline and commitment to achieve success and to overcome obstacles and we need surrender to recover and let go of attachments. I realized that my never-give-up mentality was not supporting my health and I needed more balance in my life.

Never giving up allows us to know our greatest potential. Always letting go allows us to hear our inner wisdom and honor our intuition. There is a time to push and persevere and there is a time for stillness and surrender. Balance is everything.

> *"What appears to be impossible is the wall you can only see from your present stance. If you are willing to give thanks for something you want before you see it, you will not be disappointed. Be constant to your goals, show gratitude – and one day you will look back and wonder why you ever doubted."*
>
> *– Joyce Sequichie Hifler*

Do Hard Things

Why are Spartan and Tough Mudder obstacle course endurance races so popular? What is it about climbing Mt. Everest or completing a marathon that is so inspiring? What moment in your life did you feel most proud and empowered? Why is it that doing hard things, overcoming adversity and conquering fears and obstacles makes us feel so alive? I think it's a combination of adrenaline and the sense of accomplishment that lights us up.

A book called *"Do Hard Things: A Teenage Rebellion Against Low Expectations"* was written by twin teen brothers whose vision was to start an inspiring movement against low expectations in young people. I love the concept and mission of this book and admire its writers for encouraging our youth to get out of their comfort zone and challenge themselves in life.

There are plenty of people who always take the easy route. Just as many people choose to do hard things because even though the challenge is scary, the independence and rewards outweigh the difficulties. The high you get from facing fear and doing it anyway is unlike any high you can get from a drug and it's equally addictive.

Some of the most rewarding moments of my life happened when I stepped out of my comfort zone. Going on a two-week adventure to India with YogaFit was both challenging and transformational. Volunteering at Knights of Heroes camp to mentor children who lost their fathers in service to our country was emotional and exhausting, but rewarding beyond measure.

One of the biggest challenges of my life came unexpectedly when my brother died in a car accident. Losing him led me to go to India, which had been on my bucket list for years, and to volunteer at the Knights of Heroes camp with my nephew and my husband. Although a tragedy led me there, I am grateful for the experiences I had with both of these outstanding organizations. These challenges taught me the valuable quality of how to be more comfortable being uncomfortable.

My brother, Scott, had his willpower tested when he went through Marine Corps boot camp at Parris Island, SC in 1983. His graduation day was one of the proudest moments of his life. Why? Because boot camp was hard and because he earned it.

Although his willpower was tested, he also learned to be mentally flexible in ways I couldn't comprehend. He could sleep anywhere, would eat anything and would give you the shirt off his back without question. He'd break or sprain a limb, gash his leg, be sick with the flu, or all of the above and he never complained. I don't know if boot camp taught him that or if that was just the way he was.

Before being diagnosed with Type 1 diabetes, he lost 30 pounds in a few weeks and wasn't feeling well for months. He kept it to himself, until I saw him one day and gasped at how bad he looked. I forced him to go to the hospital. His blood sugar was so high, it was literally off the charts. I remember the doctor telling me that the gash in his leg had gotten infected with staph, which likely caused his immune system to go on full alert. Since the infection was left untreated, it eventually caused an autoimmune reaction, leading to his Type 1 diabetes. At the time, I didn't understand. Many years later, a doctor told me that my untreated Lyme infection likely caused my autoimmune thyroid disease.

My brother's ability to block out discomfort and not complain was admirable, but it put his health at serious risk. Sometimes doing hard things can put us in danger. Although he may not have been the most physically flexible guy, Scott was mentally flexible, as I believe most military service men and women are. They have to be! They are put into situations that would crush most of us.

While willpower, never giving up and doing hard things are essential for success, chillpower, surrendering and doing easy things allows us to be more resilient and bend without breaking. It's the balance of these two opposites that connects us to our greatest warrior strength.

"Going too far is as bad as falling short."

 – **Chinese Proverb**

*"If you listen to your body when it whispers,
you won't have to hear it scream."*

 – **Indian Proverb**

*"Train yourself to let go of everything you
fear to lose."*

 – **Yoda, Star Wars**

2

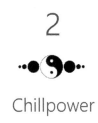

Chillpower

A Flexible Warrior is both strong and resilient. Your powerful and focused willpower can benefit greatly from its relaxed and flexible opposite, chillpower. For people with a never-give-up mentality, it's hard to feel good about surrendering. How can you stay true to your work ethic and values while letting go?

Chillpower, like anything worthwhile, takes practice. Like willpower, once you feel the benefits it can be addictive as well as contagious. Anyone who has ever sought out a yoga class has plugged-in to the contagious power of peace.

In the beginning, it may be awkward or even stressful to just sit and breathe. Surrender can bring a sense of discomfort and vulnerability. It might feel depressing to let go of a goal or to ask for help. Even strong warriors and superheroes need support. With faith and an open mind, we can begin to see the new opportunities, peace and power that come with letting go when the time is right. The key is knowing when to push harder and when to pull back. If you surrender too soon you might miss an opportunity. Once you've gone over the edge, it's too late and there is usually a hefty price to pay at that point, whether it be injury, chronic illness, or even a destroyed relationship. Have the confidence to be authentic and true to yourself despite what others think. Trust your intuition to guide you.

Understanding the balance between Abhyasa (never give up) and Vairagya (always let go) can bring much power and peace.

Less is More

Yoga is a perfect example of how less can be more. If you push into a stretch or try to muscle through a yoga class, not only is it unenjoyable, it also backfires. When you force or struggle in a stretch, you'll actually get tighter and more tense. This stretch reflex is your body's natural protective response to keep you from injuries caused by overstretching. Taking a slow, gentle approach to stretching is how you get your body to relax and open up. It's like a flower in a tight bud. If you try to force it open, it destroys the process. When the flower unfolds naturally, it's perfect and beautiful. A less-is-more approach to stretching allows you to relax, accept where you are and let nature takes its course. Doing less doesn't mean not trying. It just means not forcing.

I also notice that the less clutter, stress and drama I have in my life, the more clarity, peace and joy I experience. I don't buy a lot of material things. I don't fill my house with clutter or surround myself with drama. I donate frequently to clear out whatever I don't need and I let go of toxic relationships. The more I do these things, the happier I am.

Yoga has a reputation of being easy, but many styles of yoga are very challenging, especially for newcomers. What's easy for one person can be hard for another. Too much of a good thing can also cause imbalance and problems. Being too flexible, physically or mentally, can get us in trouble. Overstretching can lead to joint instability and injury. Being too mentally flexible can lead to being a doormat and never doing what you want when you want. The less-is-more approach will benefit you in a yoga practice, but also many other areas of life. As you do hard things, strive for a healthy, balanced sense of mental and physical flexibility.

A close friend of mine, Jimmy Page, co-wrote a book called *One Word That Will Change Your Life.* This book has helped me apply the less-is-more concept to my daily life. Instead of new year resolutions and lists of goals, I choose one single word that reflects how I want to feel and the general direction I want to head. I use this one word as my compass when I set my daily intentions. Discovering the power of "One Word" has helped me experience more simplicity and focus and live with more passion, power and purpose.

"One Word has helped me focus less on what I was doing and more on who I was becoming."

– Jimmy Page, author, speaker and VP for Fellowship of Christian Athletes

Applying the less-is-more approach to fitness can be beneficial too. I have a good friend, Gaby, who is a disciplined and dedicated runner. The year her mom died she trained for her first marathon. It was very inspiring to watch her run in her mom's honor and raise money for cancer research.

Gaby caught the marathon bug and ran a few more half marathons the following year. She trained with a coached group and followed all the rules, except for one. She logged all her weekly mileage and progressively built her distance and pace, but would consistently skip her cross training and recovery days in order to log more miles.

Even though Gaby is a yoga and stretching enthusiast, she felt like running more would help her be a better runner. It seemed logical! But after about a year, she began having a dull pain. She invested in expensive running shoes, saw a sports medicine doctor, a chiropractor and a physical therapist and was diagnosed with spinal (lumbar and sacral) stenosis with bulges in two discs, leading to sciatica.

Despite the annoying pain, she kept running and logging lots of miles. Soon enough, the repetitive motion led to extreme pain and she had to take months off. She then realized that if she had run less, rested more and listened to her body when the twinges started, she would have saved herself a lot of time, money and pain. She didn't need fancy shoes. She needed rest!

The interesting thing is that Gaby is more mindful and balanced than the average Jane. But there is something so addictive about training for races and exercise in general that it brainwashes us into thinking that more is more. In reality, being 10-15 percent undertrained is more effective than being over-trained and sidelined with an overuse injury.

When you skip cross training, flexibility and recovery in order to pound your body more, it's counterproductive and potentially destructive. Gaby's term for this ineffective training is 'junk miles', which is a waste of your valuable training time. Consider taking a less-is-more approach to your training and enjoy your recovery days knowing that it will make you stronger and more resilient.

Award for Most Grateful

I'm not a fast runner. For a blip in time on my middle school and high school track teams I was relatively fast. I say "relatively" because there wasn't much competition in my small Pennsylvania town. The joy of passing people and running fast was exhilarating while it lasted. I would love to go back in time and experience that again. However, around the age of 16, I noticed others were zipping by me in the sprints.

In the summer of 2009, I trained for the Irongirl sprint distance triathlon in Columbia, Maryland. At the finish line, a spectator told me I should win an award for smiling the most. He said most of the women he saw racing were so serious, but he appreciated that I was thanking everyone, waving and smiling.

The next year, I cheered on a few of my friends who raced. They were all smiling and waving too. None of us won an award for speed, but it occurred to me that there should be an award for 'Most Grateful' and more encouragement to slow down and enjoy the journey instead of criticizing ourselves for not being faster. Just finishing is a huge accomplishment! I feel it's important and uplifting to take the time along the way to thank the volunteers who gave up their Saturday to support us, the police officers who protect us and the cheerleaders, friends and family who encourage us. After a race I like to do "legs up the wall" pose and send gratitude to my legs for carrying me.

There are plenty of true athletes who train hard and deserve to go full speed ahead. I honor their spirit and try to stay out of their way. One day I'd like to create my own yoga-inspired race that's more about gratitude than speed. I'll call it the Flexible Warrior Chillpower Run. We'll start with superfoods, breathing and Sun Salutations, run at our own enjoyable pace and finish with gentle yoga stretches, green smoothies, meditation, a lavender spritz and a long Savasana (relaxation). Who's in? There will definitely be gratitude medals and wheat grass shots when you cross the finish line.

Warriors in battle sacrifice and conquer with strength and determination. Adrenaline kicks in, the fight or flight instinct takes over and nothing is impossible. Even with injuries or what seems like insurmountable obstacles, a warrior single-mindedly pursues his or her goal. We see it all the time in real life and in inspiring movies like *Star Wars* and *Braveheart* to Disney movies like *The Lion King* and *Brave*. Heroic acts are always inspiring.

In our day-to-day life, we don't need to approach it like it's a live-or-die battle scene. Mental toughness and willpower can accomplish amazing things, but so can flexibility and chillpower.

It's easy to get on a downward spiral when we have an injury or illness and feel that our bodies are fighting us or that life is unfair and that we aren't getting what we want and deserve. It's hard to believe that letting go is exactly the thing that will open us up to new possibility.

I learned about the power of surrender from fighting an autoimmune disease. Your teacher might be an injury or obstacle of another kind. For years I refused to listen to my body. Fighting only made matters worse. In yoga, we learn that our obstacles and enemies are our greatest teachers. Once I embraced my situation and disease, made some lifestyle changes and let go of what was no longer serving me, my healing began. Is your body trying to tell you something? The challenges are there for a reason and our job is to listen, learn, stretch, grow and open our minds up to something greater.

Learning about Vairagya was a "light bulb" moment for me. I wasn't going with the flow at the time. I needed a new perspective. Can you relate? Have you ever experienced a time in your life when you were swimming against the current, holding onto something with a death grip and your tough, strict, bullheadedness held you back rather than allowing you to move ahead?

Maybe you know someone who is an extreme over-achiever. These warriors accomplish great things, but sometimes sacrifice relationships, their body or their sanity. Or maybe you know someone who always gives up to the point that they never accomplish a goal. These people often sacrifice their health and confidence. Neither extreme is ideal. We must find the balance point where we challenge ourselves and achieve great things, but are also able to let go when the time is right.

Staying mentally flexible when we're sidelined with an injury is tough. As crushing as it is to the mind, it can be even more crushing to the spirit. The movie *We Are Marshall* is a great example of overcoming adversity and getting back up after being knocked down.

> *"One of the hardest decisions you'll ever face in life is choosing whether to walk away or try harder."*
>
> **– idlehearts.com**

In an emotional locker room scene, star cornerback Nate Ruffin tries to persuade his coach to let him play despite a major shoulder injury. His tenacity demonstrates his willpower and willingness to do hard things. He doesn't want to give up. Nate keeps repeating, "my shoulder is fine, my shoulder is fine" in an attempt to convince himself and his coach that he could play. Despite the injury and pain, Nate did not want to surrender.

His coach replies, "I'm not questioning your courage or drive." For many athletes, surrendering to an injury is giving up. A good coach can help us see our strengths and encourage us to push our edge, yet also help us to let go when it's time to surrender. In letting go, Nate learned he could inspire, coach and assist from the sidelines while cheering his teammates on to their greatest victory.

Non-attachment is a key component of Vairagya. Letting go of goals and aspirations or even material possessions is one thing. Letting go of someone you love is another story. Ultimately the joy and experience of love is worth the pain of enduring loss. We can't let the fear of losing keep us from loving. We shouldn't let the fear and embarrassment of failure keep us from trying. Peace comes with trusting we are safe and are exactly where we are meant to be.

> *"Some of us think holding on makes us strong but sometimes it is letting go."*
>
> **– Hermann Hesse**

Do Easy Things

Have you ever felt like you were in "the zone"? The zone feels effortless and like you are going with the flow at a pace that feels smooth and right. You can feel "in the zone" in a relationship, a race, or anytime when you're in the right place with the right people at the right time. The zone is peaceful, enjoyable and gives you a sense that you're exactly where you're supposed to be, doing exactly what you're supposed to do.

The point is that it doesn't always need to be hard to be rewarding and right! Taking the time to enjoy some easy, fun, relaxing things will make you even stronger, more energized and enthusiastic. When the time comes to do hard things you'll be ready instead of burned out.

Remember that rest, recovery and sleep are magical rebuilding tools that repair our tissues and they are as important as the training itself! Working beneath your potential and taking too much rest is lazy. Pushing over the edge and taking too little rest is destructive.

As you read through the self-care, stretching and eating ideas that follow, remember you don't have to do all of them. Take a flexible approach. Try the ones that seem the most appealing to you. Experiment and step out of your comfort zone but avoid swimming upstream. Trust your intuition and go with the flow. Give yourself permission and freedom to do easy things. See how you feel.

There is no magic one-size-fits-all solution. What works for me may not be a match for your body type, chemistry or personality. Your job is to figure out the amount of time you can commit and the particular techniques that make you feel your best.

"When health is absent,

wisdom cannot reveal itself,

art cannot manifest,

strength cannot fight,

wealth becomes useless

and intelligence cannot be applied."

– Herophilus

PART II

Protect, Stretch and Eat Like A Warrior

"I have come to believe that caring for myself is not self-indulgent. Caring for myself is an act of survival."

– Audre Lorde

"It's very important that we re-learn the art of resting and relaxing. Not only does it help prevent the onset of many illnesses that develop through chronic tension and worrying; it allows us to clear our minds, focus and find creative solutions to problems."

– Thich Nhat Hanh

"Rest and self-care are so important. When you take time to replenish your spirit, it allows you to serve others from the overflow. You cannot serve from an empty vessel."

– Eleanor Brownn

3

Self-care for Warriors

Does a massage feel like an indulgence? Does sitting still feel like a waste of time? If so, you could probably benefit from some extreme self-care.

A warrior wouldn't go into battle without a shield. An over-trained body and a stressed out mind can weaken your immune system, which is your protective shield against infection and illness. When your body is worn down, you are more prone to injury. Moderate exercise can boost immunity, but extreme exercise can decrease immune function. A little less body-wrecking and a little more self-care can create more strength and resilience.

Massage techniques can relax and loosen up tense, tight muscles. Breathing and meditation can help calm and center the mind. Healthy eating and good digestion will positively affect immune function to keep you stronger and healthier from the inside out.

Consider that some of the best self-care techniques are free: quality sleep, deep breathing and hydration. Self-care includes the spiritual, mental, physical and emotional aspects of your life. When one of these essential elements is missing, we are imbalanced.

You've heard the quote: "You can't give from an empty cup." Self-care is not self-indulgent. In fact, you are better able to take care of others when you are healthy and recharged. I believe unhealthy behaviors like smoking, eating junk foods and over-exercising can be selfish acts because they weaken you, increase the chances you'll be a burden to someone else and decrease your ability to be strong for others.

Experiment with a few of these techniques. Doing new things can be intimidating, but a warrior goes into the unknown despite the fear. You do so many hard things. See what happens when you try some nurturing, gentle, easy things. There are thousands of gifted healing hands out there waiting to help you.

I'm Flexible! Are You?

When I'm making plans and scheduling appointments, I find myself saying "I'm flexible" constantly. We are what we say we are! Flexibility is a state of mind as well as a physical benefit. I know people who say their life is "crazy" all the time. I think statements can become affirmations. Whether intentional or not, you are reinforcing beliefs with your words.

Whether it's 10 minutes before sunrise, five minutes at your lunch break or 30 minutes after dinner, setting aside a daily chunk of time to breathe and stretch is key to your success for harnessing the power of self-care and flexibility. You may not fit it in every single day and that's okay! Try to fit in one to two hours of self-care each week at minimum.

Some weeks, you could book a self-care service like a

massage or acupuncture and that session counts toward your Flexible Warrior time! If you're receiving a self-care service one day and you don't have time for anything else, you can skip your meditation or stretch session, but pick back up the following day. You're practicing being flexible mentally as well as physically. Stressing about your self-care is counterproductive. Avoid rushing to your massage appointment and leaving in a panic. Try not to worry or feel guilty during your yoga class. Dig deeper into your chillpower mindset and enjoy your rest and recovery.

Yoga Off The Mat

I once watched one of my yoga students through the studio window as she left class. She hurried out before final relaxation and rushed to her car. In the parking lot, someone cut in front of her. She freaked out, beeped her horn, yelled and flipped them off.

I also see students practicing good posture, alignment and breathing during class only to slump as they throw their heavy bag over their shoulder. The one or two hours a week of self-care are critical, but what you do with the rest of your 168 hours is even more important.

There is a term we yogis call "yoga off the mat" which means what we do on our mat needs to carry off our mat and into our lives. Practice being flexible, aligned and balanced in everything you do including how you eat, how you act and how you interact in all your relationships. Let your self-care spill over and positively affect your entire life. Instead of coming from a depleted place, fill your self-care cup up so full that you have plenty to share with others.

Loosening Up Tin Man

If you wake up in the morning feeling stiff and tight, you are not alone! Chronic tension is common, especially as we age. You can reduce and possibly eliminate the stiffness and pain by incorporating a healing anti-inflammatory diet along with a regular self-massage and stretching practice.

After Lyme, I was chronically achy, stiff, sore and tight. My personal mission was to get my muscles and body out of pain without drugs. It wasn't easy and I still have flare ups on occasion, especially when I'm stressed and don't practice enough self-care. Ironically, writing this book has caused me to skip my regular routine and has served as a gentle reminder not to sacrifice my self-care.

If you'd like to sleep better and wake up energized and pain-free, realize that, like all training, it takes commitment, practice, patience and consistency. You have to be willing to put the time in to get the results.

As you experiment with the different techniques, take note of the one to three that really work for you, fit your personality, goals, budget and schedule. Make them non-negotiables that you commit to daily, weekly or monthly. Do a three month trial and see how you feel. Add self-care and flexibility to your training schedule. Put it on your calendar to make it a priority.

There have been many times I wished I had a magic wand to wave over my clients to instantly heal them. What I've discovered is that the most powerful healing comes from quality food and investing in self-care. Most medications don't heal. They often just mask symptoms and create side effects that can often make matters worse. The transformation that comes from changing your diet and making better lifestyle choices is very empowering.

Chronic Inflammation Versus Acute Inflammation

Before we get into the self-care techniques, let's discuss the difference between chronic and acute inflammation. Information about inflammation is everywhere these days. But, when I was diagnosed with autoimmune disease it was not even on the radar, at least not with my doctors. Our knowledge is evolving constantly and this gives us all opportunities to improve our health with the lifestyle and food choices we make rather than using medications alone.

Acute inflammation is your body's natural response to heal an injury or fight an infection, like if you sprain your ankle or have the flu. If you've had swelling from an injury or a fever from an illness, you have experienced acute inflammation. The beauty is you don't have to tell your body to do anything. The healing kicks in automatically and little warrior cells within you go to battle to repair you.

The recovery time may feel like it is passing slowly during the rebuild phase, but before you know it you're back to normal. Isn't it miraculous what the body can do? The healing process is not unlike recovery from hard training. The good stress of exercise creates microscopic tears in your muscles, called micro trauma, which then swell with blood in order to repair and grow stronger. Acute inflammation is a powerful, good and healthy process! The healthier you are, the faster and more efficient the repair process will happen. That should be motivation enough to practice self-care and eat well.

Think of it this way. If you were renovating your house and had to choose between Team A: the strong, fast, healthy, fit, efficient guys who get the job done right and on time, or Team B: the guys that sleep in, live on coffee, cigarettes and donuts, don't sleep well and end up behind schedule and sloppy... which team would you choose? It's the same with your immune system. Keep your internal warrior cells healthy, well-rested and well-fed and they will be ready to go to battle at a moment's notice. They'll repair you quickly if you're in an accident or are exposed to a virus.

Chronic inflammation is more complicated. When we are exposed to a lot of environmental toxins, junk foods, unhealthy habits like smoking or drinking too much alcohol, or even over-exercising, our bodies and our immune system can wear down, rebel and create a chronic inflammatory response.

Chronic inflammation is sometimes subtle. Symptoms can be headaches, stiff achy joints, allergies, arthritis, autoimmune diseases, rashes, fatigue, digestive issues and even acne, just to name a few. Your doctor might prescribe antidepressants or anti-inflammatories to mask the symptoms. These medications can't fix the root cause, which can be partly genetic, but are also influenced by stress, toxins, infections and of course diet. While months of antibiotics improved my Lyme symptoms, changing my diet took my healing to a whole new level.

My autoimmune trigger was Lyme. Since I couldn't go back in time and eliminate the tick bite that caused the disease, reducing stress and my exposure to toxins, along with changing my diet, was essential for my immune system's recovery. The same anti-inflammatory diet that prevents and heals autoimmunity also prevents and heals most other diseases. Reducing inflammation improves healing from other trauma, like sports injuries, and helps to decrease joint and muscle stiffness from arthritis and fibromyalgia.

A lot of people take prescription or over the counter drugs daily to keep the chronic pain and inflammation at bay. But an anti-inflammatory diet can help reduce pain and stiffness naturally and the only side effect is you will feel great, be healthier and feel more resilient and flexible!

Chronic inflammation was once described to me in a way that really got my attention: if you're standing on a tack and it's digging into your heel, you could take painkillers to numb the ache and anti-inflammatories to reduce the swelling or you could just step off the tack and let your body heal! When given a chance, your body can and will repair itself. The symptoms of pain and stiffness are not the enemy. They are the messenger telling us something needs to change. Are you willing to do what it takes to let your body heal?

For a healthy immune system and balanced inflammatory response: Exercise, not too much, not too little. Eat well. Sleep well. Stretch and relax. And, if you have a tack in your foot, pull it out!

Massage

Healing touch has been around since the beginning of time. But as with doctors, lawyers and even yoga teachers, there are good ones and not so good ones. A gifted massage therapist who uses the power of touch with a positive intention has amazing healing powers. However, there are others that are unfocused, uncaring, uneducated or are doing it for all the wrong reasons. A bad massage is a waste of your precious time and money.

I've only experienced a bad massage once in my life and I swore afterward that I'd only book with a referral. You deserve someone fantastic and passionate who understands, cares and knows your body. Ask around and schedule regular appointments with a good massage therapist. Also, make sure your masseuse practices self-care so when they work on you they are coming from a good, grounded place.

There are a lot of different massage styles: deep tissue,

Swedish, Rolfing, Shiatsu, aromatherapy and hot stone massage, just to name a few. Experiment and find what you like. Think of it more as maintenance. It's better to get your oil changed and stay on top of your car service rather than waiting until after you have a breakdown. Don't take better care of your car than yourself!

Consider having your massage therapist use magnesium oil and/or coconut oil for your massage. I take mine with me and have the massage therapist use it instead of their standard massage oil, which can often be full of toxins. Magnesium is a natural muscle relaxant. Coconut oil is moisturizing and great for your skin. Don't shower these healthy oils off right away. Let them soak into your skin all day and night while sleeping. Just be aware the magnesium oil can feel a little tingly, so it might not be the most relaxing for a massage, especially if your skin is sensitive. Test it out first.

Massage can increase circulation and help to speed healing. Incorporating self-care has helped me prevent and shorten the frequency of my autoimmune flare ups, but hasn't altogether eliminated them. Bear in mind, depending on your particular issue, you must give your body time to heal at its own pace.

Reiki

Reiki is a Japanese technique that's great for reducing stress and increasing relaxation. The touch is very light or hovers above your skin. For many people, Reiki can be more relaxing and more healing than massage. Some practitioners combine massage with Reiki techniques, which is a wonderful way to get the healing benefits of both styles. I always leave a Reiki session feeling light, energized and more aligned in mind, body and spirit.

In my experience, someone who has been trained in Reiki is very in tune with how others are feeling and they have a very healing, almost magical touch. No matter what service or body work you're receiving, it's all about the practitioner's energy and intention as well as you, the receiver, being open. If you're new to Reiki, consider trying a session that combines massage with Reiki energy work to get a sense of how it makes you feel.

Magnesium and Alternative Pain Relief Creams

Many people are low in minerals like magnesium. This is partly due to poor diet but is also because the soil we grow our vegetables in is depleted of minerals due to over-farming. Even if you're eating lots of veggies, you might still not be getting enough magnesium. Being low in this mineral can cause muscle cramping, general soreness and fatigue.

Magnesium is a natural muscle relaxant. Topical magnesium lotion or oil is absorbed transdermally, through your skin. Using it before bedtime or with body work such as massage or foam rolling can be very healing. If your skin is sensitive to the magnesium, try it on your feet since the skin is tougher there.

As grateful as I am for modern medicine, I'd rather endure a little discomfort than pop a pill for every ache. Pain is an important messenger communicating to us. If we always dull our sensation with a drug, then we are less likely to clearly hear the message.

I have had issues with chronic headaches for as long as I can remember. I medicated myself for years with migraine drugs and other painkillers. What I discovered works better for me than any drug (with no side effects) is a huge glass of water, magnesium (I use Natural Calm and Ancient Minerals) yoga and a nap. Headaches are often a sign of dehydration, a mineral deficiency or fatigue.

Magnesium is responsible for over 300 biomechanical functions in the body, so a lot can go wrong when there is a deficiency. My source of all things magnesium is Dr. Carolyn Dean. Although she has no idea who I am, I am forever grateful for the information she shares on her blog and e-newsletters.

Other alternative pain relief creams include Arnica and Traumeel. Arnica is made from an herb and is used for bruises, aches and pains. Traumeel is a homeopathic remedy used to help reduce pain and inflammation.

Acupuncture and Dry Needling

These two techniques are different yet the results I got from both were similar. Based in Chinese medicine, acupuncture involves a practitioner inserting very thin needles into the skin to stimulate specific meridian points on the body. Acupuncture is great for treating pain and injuries, but it's also wonderful for treating illness, disease and general well-being. Acupuncture can help with pretty much anything from quitting smoking to getting pregnant!

I was first exposed to acupuncture while I was being treated for Lyme disease. Although it was expensive, part of it was covered by my insurance. It was a big commitment of my time and money, but I decided to go once or twice a week for six weeks to see if it would help.

I became a believer after my first week. Once the needles were inserted, I'd lie there and meditate, imagining the healing happening in my body or listening to a guided imagery CD. The combination of acupuncture and meditation can be very effective. It's rare to lie still for 30 to 60 minutes, so why not make the most productive use of that time!

In later years, I saw a physical therapist for chronic neck pain and headaches. In addition to exercises and stretches, he incorporated dry needling, a similar technique to acupuncture that is used to treat muscle pain. I had good results from dry needling as well. But like all self-care techniques, it's important to stay consistent, to incorporate lifestyle changes and to figure out the triggers and the root causes of your pain.

As with all services, the practitioner's touch, style, intention and education can make a huge difference. Do your research and ask around to get a referral for an acupuncturist or physical therapist.

Hot Bath with Epsom Salts

A hot bath is one of the cheapest, most convenient self-care techniques and it can be very effective! A 20 to 30 minute soak in a hot bath, especially when you add mineral-rich Epsom salts and some essential oils, feels great, reduces stress, relaxes muscles and boosts immunity and overall health.

A hot bath can help you sleep better, alleviate fatigue, increase blood flow and reduce inflammation. You might be surprised at how this simple, inexpensive, old school secret really makes a difference! One of the reasons Epsom salt is so helpful in relaxing sore, tight muscles is that it's high in magnesium. If you don't have access to a big bathtub or don't have time to soak for 30 minutes, try magnesium oil or lotion instead.

Ice Bath/Contrast Therapy

An ice bath isn't as relaxing as a hot bath, but it's used often in sports therapy after intense training to reduce pain and swelling. Contrast therapy alternates between hot and cold and certainly fits into our "balance of opposites" theme. There is a lot of controversy over the effectiveness and safety of these techniques, but the Flexible Warrior principle applies (we'll cover that more in Chapter 4). When it comes to matters of self-care, if it feels good and it works for you, do it!

My muscles don't respond well to cold, so I don't have a lot of personal experience with the cold tub or contrast therapy. One winter, though, I was on vacation in Mexico and I decided to participate in an ancient ritual that involved sitting in a little pitch black cave-like sauna for 30 minutes followed by an ice-cold plunge. It was exhilarating to say the least.

I know athletes who relax in a sauna or a steam room and follow with a dip in a cold tub. Others do intervals of hot and cold in the shower or alternate using ice packs with a heating pad to create the hot/cold contrast therapy. In the end, I think it's about increasing circulation and generating healing blood flow to the tissues.

Inflammation is a healthy and important part of healing and repair. Be aware that some studies have shown that icing an injury, which reduces pain and swelling temporarily, can slow down the healing process. The body's natural healing process creates inflammation and heat by increasing circulation to the injured area, which is why there is swelling and redness. The body knows what it is doing! Those who oppose icing feel that you can potentially slow healing by interfering. Talk to your doctor or physical therapist to decide what's best for you.

Thai Massage

Thai massage originated in Thailand and is often called Thai Yoga. Some people say it feels like yoga, but without the effort. You just lie there and are manually assisted into stretches and poses. You wear comfortable yoga-type clothes and lie on a big, cushy mat on the floor for a Thai massage. The therapist will work pressure points in your body using both their hands and feet for the poses, stretches and massage.

Thai massage is one of those experiences you need to try in order to completely understand and appreciate. It's a little harder to find than a regular Swedish or sports massage, but there are practitioners in most major cities and at some spas.

If you're fairly inflexible and don't stretch often, a Thai massage can be a little intimidating. Like all massage, communicate with your practitioner. If you have a thing about feet, just know that someone's feet will be all over you. But if you have an issue with getting naked for a traditional massage, Thai Massage may be worth checking out, since you stay fully clothed.

Receiving any kind of bodywork can feel intimate and awkward if you overthink it, but when you relax your mind and let go, receiving the healing touch from someone who truly cares can open up places in your body and bring a sense of ease, relaxation and healing.

I'm trained in Thai Massage, so I may be a little biased. To me it's a wonderful combo of massage, stretching and yoga. If you want a completely different massage experience with some assisted stretching, a Thai Massage should be on your list.

Reflexology/Self-Foot Massage

When something goes wrong with your feet, it can affect the whole body so taking care of your precious foundation is essential. Most of us pound our feet into the pavement and cram them into fashionable shoes without a thought. Anyone who has ever had plantar fasciitis or a broken toe can attest to how much your feet matter. We often don't really value our feet until we have a problem.

Reflexology is not just a foot massage. It gives attention to the hands as well and it involves pressure points that correspond with all areas of the body, including organs. It's great for general, as well as, foot health.

One summer while I was training for a 10K, I got plantar fasciitis, a painful inflammation of the heel and underside of the foot. I had been running and stretching regularly and feeling great, until one day I stepped on a nail in the center of my heel and ran later that day. After that, I had severe heel pain for months. I took three months off from running and during that time I invested in six weekly reflexology sessions. In addition, I was rolling my feet on a frozen water bottle, doing self-massage with a tennis ball (although I now prefer Jill Miller's Yoga Tune Up balls), stretching, acupuncture, yoga and I wore the dreaded night splint brace.

What I can say for sure is that reflexology felt great and after three months my foot got better! But since I combined it with so many other techniques, I can't be positive of its effect on my healing. The pain eventually dissolved completely and I was back to running with no problems.

Take care of your feet and try reflexology. Many massage therapists are also trained in foot massage techniques so, when you book your next massage, ask for extra attention on your feet and see how you feel.

Self-Massage/Myofascial Release

There is nothing like a hands-on massage to reduce stress and induce relaxation and healing. Combining self-massage with your regular self-care is a very effective complement to create longer lasting effects. With a few inexpensive tools, self- massage is free, convenient and with consistency, can reduce pain and improve flexibility!

Fascia is the connective tissue that surrounds muscle, bones and ligaments. It lies under our skin, above our muscles and covers our whole body from head to toe like a sheath of saran wrap. The more trauma your body endures, the more fascia layers it will create, which can eventually cause pain and reduced range of motion.

Trigger points are tender knots in the fascia or tight bands of muscle fibers that can cause a lot of pain, including referred pain to other areas of the body. Issues with fascia and trigger points can be caused by over-training, dehydration, poor nutrition, inadequate recovery, lack of quality sleep, or even trauma from a car accident.

Since self-massage relaxes muscles and increases blood flow, I find that foam rolling before stretching enhances flexibility training. The good news is our fascial system, like our muscles and organs, is very adaptable and can improve with consistent flexibility work. But it will also get tighter and more restricted depending on how we move and fuel our bodies. The more repetitive and stressful our activities are and the more sugar and inflammatory foods we eat, the thicker and less resilient the fascia becomes. People think that stiffness naturally comes with age, but it doesn't have to be that way.

Inflammatory foods have an effect on the health of all our tissue including fascia. For more pliable, resilient fascia, eat clean, whole foods that emphasize lean proteins, Omega-3 fatty acids, fruits and vegetables, all of which have anti-inflammatory properties. Minimize sugar, alcohol and processed foods.

Self-massage tools I love include: The Stick, a high density foam roller, the TriggerPoint Therapy GRID Roller and Therapy massage balls, the Posture Ball by OTPT and Jill Miller's Yoga Tune Up Therapy balls. Also check out MobilityWOD for great content on reducing pain and increasing flexibility.

Ki-Hara/Mashing

I was watching swimmer Dara Torres in awe during the 2008 summer Olympics. She and I are close in age so I was inspired by her strength, speed and incredible physique. During an Olympic feature segment, they showed Dara getting stretched by two trainers before her competition. I had been teaching yoga and Spinning for the Baltimore Ravens football team for a few consecutive seasons so I was always looking for flexibility routines for the players. Dara and her stretchers had my complete attention.

After some research, I discovered the method Dara used to stretch was called Ki-Hara and was taught by Steven Sierra and Anne Tierney (the two stretchers that traveled to the Olympics with Dara). A few months later, I was taking a Ki-Hara training with Steve and Anne.

I had been teaching yoga and stretching for years, but this training technique made me feel things I had never felt before in my body. I was hooked. To add to my enthusiasm, both Anne and Steve were so smart and charismatic that I felt compelled to pursue the Ki-Hara training further. At the training I met Susan Bianchi, one of the Ki-Hara master trainers, and began an internship with her.

What is Ki-Hara?

Most traditional styles of stretching, including yoga, are static in nature, where you hold a stretch in a lengthened position for 30-60 seconds. Ki-Hara incorporates resistance stretching, where a trainer assists and slightly resists the client throughout a range of motion during the stretch. The result is strength with flexibility throughout an entire range of motion. It's the ultimate stability with mobility. Trust me, it's good stuff.

> *"Remember it is not how far your body (and mind) can lengthen or stretch but that there is strength throughout your range. Without that strength, we are susceptible to injury. Being flexible requires having strength throughout the movement in order to be resilient, to bounce back physically and mentally."*
>
> **– Susan Bianchi, Ki-Hara Master Trainer and owner of Intrinsic Health Systems**

An important part of Ki-Hara is "mashing," a form of bodywork where practitioners use their feet to compress and massage the client. The mashing technique is so effective that I've had NFL players, Ironman distance triathletes, marathon runners, CrossFit competitors and an Olympian book 90 minute mash-only sessions to help them recover faster. Mashing looks weird but it feels great. It's a combination of a Thai Massage, Shiatsu and deep tissue massage. Practitioners use their feet to work on fascia, loosen up muscles and flush toxins before and after the resistance stretches. The advantage of using feet instead of hands is that you can get deeper into the tissue. Many practitioners even use a granny walker to stabilize as they walk all over people. It's an interesting and effective technique. I highly recommend you seek out a Ki-Hara trainer in your area and give it a try!

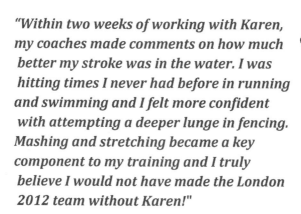

"Working with Karen and her mashing treatments have been pivotal to my career. I'm in my 13th year as a professional football player and I wouldn't be able to play at such a high level without her."

- Terrell Suggs, Ravens linebacker and six-time Pro Bowler

"Within two weeks of working with Karen, my coaches made comments on how much better my stroke was in the water. I was hitting times I never had before in running and swimming and I felt more confident with attempting a deeper lunge in fencing. Mashing and stretching became a key component to my training and I truly believe I would not have made the London 2012 team without Karen!"

– Suzanne Stettinius, Olympian

Chiropractic Adjustments & Physical Therapy

Yes, physical therapy is mentioned twice because over the years, I've seen many different types of PTs and they all have a unique approach. If you've tried one and didn't get the results you wanted, try someone else! That rule applies to chiropractors, to all bodyworkers and to yoga teachers as well as pretty much everything in life. The hardest part is having the tenacity to try again. It's like dating and finding "the one." Don't settle for average.

The musculoskeletal and musculature system is complex. A good chiropractor can perform adjustments and manipulate the spine and other parts of the body to bring it into better alignment. A good physical therapist can teach you exercises and stretches that can help you improve movement and reduce pain.

It can be expensive and time consuming to keep up with self-care services. Commitment is key, so whatever you decide to do, give it a chance and commit for a period of time. You can't go just once and hope to be magically cured of all pain. Like all training, if you want results, you need repetition and consistency. For athletes and anyone suffering with musculoskeletal issues, chiropractic adjustments and physical therapy can both be very worthwhile.

Sleep

According to the CDC, 50 to 70 million American adults have sleep disorders. Not getting enough sleep is linked to a long list of mental and physical health problems, including an increase in the frequency of common colds and flu viruses and, consequently, decreased performance and more sick days.

Quality sleep is absolutely #1 when it comes to

strengthening our shield. No matter if you are a high level athlete or a stay-at-home mom, when sleep is cut short the body doesn't have enough time to release the essential hormones to repair the body and the brain. Limited sleep raises the levels of the stress hormone cortisol, which can have many negative effects on the immune system, mind and body. It can also increase your chances of fatiguing faster, getting sick more often, having brain fog, poor energy and a lack of enthusiasm.

When you are sleep deprived you are more likely to reach for inflammatory foods like caffeine and sugar, which may temporarily give you a boost in energy, but will soon leave your mind more fatigued and your body more inflamed. Our diet and stretching choices can be based on preference, but we all need sleep. Little things can make a big difference in the length and quality of your sleep: disconnecting from electronic devices one to two hours before bedtime, hydrating earlier in the day and cutting back on liquids after dinner. Also, skipping caffeine after 2PM, investing in room darkening shades and sticking to a regular sleep schedule can help. Make quality sleep a priority!

Hydration

What does hydration have to do with flexibility, immunity and self-care? Everything! Dehydration is chronic in our culture due to exercise, medications, caffeine, environmental toxins, air conditioning and heating, travel and poor diet. Chronic dehydration can cause pain and disease.

I have many plants in my house (you know they help clean the air and oxygenate the environment, right?) but my Peace Lily is my favorite. First of all, it was given to me after my brother died, so it reminds me daily of the value of life. Secondly, it acts as a reminder of the importance of hydration. If you don't stay on top of watering a Peace Lily, it will go limp quickly. But within minutes of watering, its leaves will perk back up with life like magic.

Ninety percent of our body is water and every cell needs hydration to thrive, including our joints, connective tissue and muscles. Symptoms like fatigue and body pain are often a sign of dehydration. Instead of reaching for water, we reach for painkillers and stimulants like caffeine and sugar, which only further dehydrate. Drinking more water can flush out toxins, rehydrate tissues, improve circulation and reduce pain. Your body is able to heal itself on all levels much faster and more efficiently when it's properly hydrated. Although needs may vary depending on variables such as body weight and exercise, the 8x8 rule is easy to remember and commonly advised. Aim to drink eight 8-ounce glasses a day. There are even apps to help you stay hydrated.

> *"You're not sick; you're thirsty. Don't treat thirst with medication."*
>
> **-Dr. Batmanghelidj,**
> *The Water Cure*

Drinking plain water can be boring. Here are a few tips to rehydrate:

1) First thing in the morning, drink a huge glass of water (yes before your coffee or tea because even though they have water in them they are dehydrating!)
2) Consider swapping out your coffee or tea for a fresh green juice or a lemon water.
3) Make a fruit water to keep in your fridge (just cut up your favorite fruits, herbs or even a hydrating veggie like cucumber and let the essence flavor your water). Some of my favorites are cucumber mint, lemon ginger and rosemary watermelon, but you can make up your own or check Pinterest for ideas.)

4) Eat your water. Especially during the hot summer months, make a point to eat more hydrating foods like cucumber, watermelon and salads.
5) Drink most of your fluids before 2PM so your sleep won't be disturbed with bathroom visits at night.
6) Squeeze a lemon into your water. It adds flavor and boosts hydration, plus helps to flush toxins.
7) Juicing is all the rage and can be a great way to rehydrate. Be sure to buy high quality fresh juices that aren't highly processed so nutrients are in tact.

If muscle cramping is an issue for you, dehydration and a deficiency in electrolytes and minerals can be a contributing factor. In addition, stretching and staying loose and relaxed in mind and body can help prevent, reduce and repair cramping. Foods high in electrolytes and magnesium can help like Celtic sea salt, coconut water, bananas and dark leafy greens. To reduce the frequency and intensity of muscle cramps, try a green smoothie along with some gentle yoga and self-massage.

Bio-Mat/Infrared Sauna

Most gyms and training facilities have a sauna or steam room. Saunas have been around for hundreds of years. The Bio-Mat and infrared sauna companies are newer on the market and claim that the deep-penetrating infrared rays and negative ions stimulate the body to heal from conditions like chronic pain, migraines and fatigue. A Google search will find a variety of benefits of sweating in a sauna, but my favorite studies are the ones I do myself.

Not everyone loves high heat. Some feel dizzy and weak while others feel invigorated and energized by high heat. It's all so individual and goes back to the not-so- scientific rule, "if it feels good you're doing it right."

The winter of 2014 was brutally cold for Maryland. I taught a Spinning and yoga combo class and afterwards would hit an infrared sauna for a 30-minute session. At the time, I was in the midst of cleaning up my diet and rebuilding my digestive tract. I came to look forward to those weekly sauna sessions. Incorporating meditation, using essential oils and drinking lots of water before, during and after was key. I continue to have chronic muscle pain from Lyme disease and it always gets worse in the winter. But during the three months that I ate a clean, anti-inflammatory diet and did the infrared sauna I felt fantastic. No flare ups!

When I first heard about the Bio-Mat I was skeptical. But I decided to give it a try, to see if it would help with my headaches and muscle pain. As a yoga teacher, my philosophy is that our injuries and illnesses are not our enemies, but rather our greatest teachers. If we use the pain or injury as an opportunity to listen to what our body is communicating to us, then we can create a new path to healing. With this principle in mind, I will share this slightly embarrassing story that opened my mind to the Bio-Mat.

I tweaked my knee on an 8K race for which I hadn't properly trained or warmed up. About 4 miles into this hilly 5-mile course, my right knee had a sharp pain so severe that I walked about a quarter mile (I'm a slow runner so my only goal is to not walk during a race). I rarely get injured since I keep all my workouts fairly moderate and practice yoga regularly. Tweaking my knee during a race was a first for me.

After crossing the finish line, I could barely walk. I limped to the car, went home, showered and followed my own advice... ice, heat, Topricin, magnesium, stretching, foam rolling and self-massage. I then hobbled to my health coach's shop to lie on her Bio-Mat for an hour. In addition, I took MSM supplements (which help with pain and inflammation) and drank a lot of water, green tea and a huge anti-inflammatory green smoothie.

This may sound completely unrelated to my run and my knee injury, but I'm one of those people who is a believer. I believe things happen for a reason. I also believe that our actions, willpower, chillpower, commitment and work ethic are what create opportunity and change. I believe that when something doesn't go the way we had hoped, or when we're faced with obstacles like injuries and illness, it's an opportunity for flexibility and resilience in action. Sometimes being a "believer" makes me vulnerable to disappointment. Other times, I think it brings me new opportunities and gifts.

You know that moment in the movie *"Signs"* when Mel Gibson says, "What kind of person are you? Do you believe in miracles? Are you the kind of person that sees signs - sees miracles? Or do you believe that people just get lucky? Is it possible that there are no coincidences?"

It might sound dramatic to compare my knee injury and Bio-Mat experience to aliens invading the planet and a wife's final words before dying after a tragic car accident. But if you believe that things happen for a reason and that they are here to communicate something important, then you'll be better able to find solutions, hope and a new path, rather than staying stuck, depressed, frustrated and pitiful on an old path that no longer serves you. In addition, believing is an important part of the placebo effect. Who cares if something is proven to work or not. If it works for you, it works!

I focused on self-care for 48 hours, realizing I'd have to cancel my clients for the week. By Monday, I was 90 percent recovered and was able to go about my day as planned. By Tuesday, I was 100 percent healed. I didn't miss a beat. I was so impressed by my fast recovery that I bought a Bio-Mat to use with clients when I stretch and mash them.

Survival of the Calmest

Often it's not the strongest or fastest competitor who wins. If you can be relaxed and in control during the critical moments, that's when the magic happens. Wasting vital energy with jitters can deplete you and pull you away from your best performance. You can be super talented, strong and uber fast, but if stress and crowd noise gets the best of you, all your strength and talent may not ever be maximized when it matters most.

The parasympathetic nervous system is in charge of rest and repair. The sympathetic system is in charge of stress and the fight-or-flight response. They are opposites and keeping them in balance is critical to optimal health. Your body will have a hard time being flexible if it's stressed and uptight. Learning to breathe properly activates the parasympathetic system and induces the relaxation response in your mind and body, allowing you to be more open and resilient in stressful situations.

"Worrying is like praying for what you don't want."

– Aileen Norton

As the saying goes, the best things in life are free and many of the best techniques to harness the power of calm are no exception. Breathing exercises, yoga, meditation and prayer are all very powerful and calming. Emotional Freedom Technique (EFT) is a style of energy work that may require a little training and cost, but it can be very effective at reducing stress and pain. Although not altogether free, a rescue dog and essential oils are two of my favorite ways to get calm and stay in the moment. The small investment you'll make will pay you back in peace and love.

Yoga

The best way to get strong, flexible and calm is by practicing yoga consistently. Yoga has been around for thousands of years and brings balance to the body, mind and spirit. It combines both physical poses (asanas) that strengthen and stretch the body and breathing exercises (pranayama) which calm and center the mind.

The word "yoga" comes from the Sanskrit term *"yuj"* which means "to unite" or "to integrate." Although we are all unique, as humans, we share many similarities. A yoga practice can bring a sense of connection within our own mind and body as well as an interconnection with others and the universe. In Chapter 5, we will further discuss our uniqueness or "bio-individuality," a term developed by the founder of the Integrative Institute of Nutrition, Joshua Rosenthal. Yoga emphasizes our sameness and oneness. Aim for a balance of both, honoring the distinctive qualities that make you special, while respecting and connecting with others.

Hatha yoga is the umbrella term that all physical yoga practices fall under. There are many styles of Hatha yoga, which we'll discuss more in Chapter 4.

Breathing

When you first enter this world from your mother's womb, you take a breath. When you die, the last thing you do is exhale. Breath is clearly life. We spend so much money on gadgetry and gear from shoes, clothes and watches to monitors, trainers and equipment. Breathing is free and when harnessed, is so powerful.

Due to stress and poor posture we are a society of chest

breathers. Belly breathing uses your lung capacity fully and oxygenates your blood completely. If you watch a baby or a dog sleep, you will see their belly rise and fall and their chest barely move. You'll be able to see their ribs expand and contract gently as they surrender to sleep and natural breath. It's very peaceful and relaxed.

Deep full inhales oxygenate the blood and energize the body. Long slow exhales induce the relaxation response and activate the parasympathetic nervous system. Deep diaphragmatic breathing allows the mind and central nervous system to calm and the muscles to release tension during a stretch.

Learning how to activate the parasympathetic nervous system can allow you to challenge yourself and go at a hard pace while staying relaxed in your mind and body. This tool can have a powerful effect on how you perform under pressure. Knowing how to stay relaxed and flexible in a physically challenging moment can keep you from tightening up, which helps prevent injuries too.

Although breathing is natural and we don't have to think about it throughout the day or night, it is a unique bodily function that we can control when we want to, positively affecting our mind and body. According to some experts, nothing has a more powerful effect on health and wellness than breathing.

In yoga, the term *Pranayama* refers to breathing practice. "Prana" means life force energy and "Yama" means to control and adjust our breathing patterns. Breath control will affect how we feel physically and emotionally. Efficient, complete breathing and getting the highest exchange of oxygen into our blood increases our Prana and enhances our performance in every way.

If a breathing practice is new for you, it may take time to feel comfortable with it. The calming, balancing or energizing effects come with practice. You can practice these breathing techniques at home, buy a book or DVD, find helpful segments on Youtube, or work with a qualified yoga teacher. Most yoga classes will start or end with a Pranayama practice.

1) 4-7-8 Relaxing Breath

I learned most of my breathing exercises at yoga trainings, but this 4-7-8 technique came from a lecture by Dr. Andrew Weil for The Integrative Institute of Nutrition curriculum. It's very simple and can be practiced almost anywhere. It is recommended that you sit up straight and place the tip of your tongue against the back of your top teeth before you start. Follow these steps:
1) To begin, exhale completely. Then inhale through your nose to a count of four
2) Hold your breath for a count of seven
3) Exhale through your mouth to a count of eight

These three steps count as one breath cycle. Complete the cycle three more times for a total of four repetitions. Lengthen your exhalations so that they take twice as long as your inhalations. This induces the relaxation response in the body, which has a calming effect on the central nervous system.

2) Ujjayi Breath

Ujjayi breath is also known as "victorious breath" and less formally as "Darth Vader breath" or "ocean breath" because it creates an audible sound that is similar to Darth Vader or the sound of ocean waves coming into the shore and back out to the sea. This style of breathing is often taught during Hatha yoga and can be both calming and energizing, helping you stay focused and increasing your ability to endure challenging poses.

To practice Ujjayi breath, you need to breathe in and out of the nose while slightly constricting the back of your throat to make an oceanic sound. You will feel and hear your breath. Contract your abdominal muscles gently at the bottom of the exhale to squeeze all the old air out and make room for a full, diaphragmatic inhale. Breathe in and out through the nose to induce the relaxation response and harness the powerful qualities of the breath.

In some group yoga classes, students will often overly emphasize the breath, but traditionally Ujjayi Pranayama should be heard and felt by you, but not by the person on a mat next to you. The best way to learn Ujjayi Pranayama is with a yoga teacher, but there are plenty of references on Youtube you can check out.

3) Three Part Breath

You can practice this breath seated with good posture (you can sit on pillows if that's more comfortable for your hips and back); reclined on your back (Savasana/Corpse pose) or lying flat on your stomach (Crocodile pose). If seated or lying on your back, you can place one hand on your chest and the other on your stomach to notice where the breath is going, or just let your arms rest by your side with palms facing up. If you're lying on your stomach, the floor will give you feedback to feel where the breath is going.

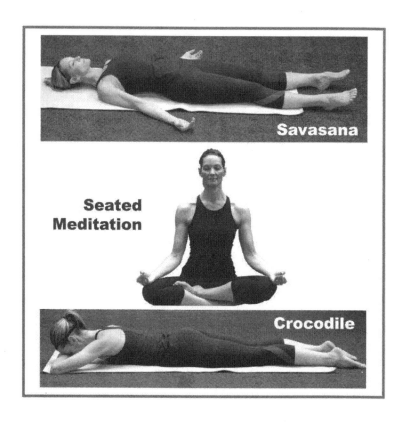

Start by closing your eyes and just observe a few breath cycles without trying to change anything. Notice if your breath is fast or slow, shallow or deep, smooth or choppy. Notice if your inhales and exhales take the same amount of time, or if the out breath is longer than the in breath. Notice if the hand on your chest or stomach is moving more. What are the qualities of your natural breathing?

Next, inhale through your nose as deeply as possible. Take the fullest breath you can, filling your lungs completely. Then exhale completely until you feel your lungs empty.

Now, focusing on the three part breath, you'll inhale again, filling your belly first, then your ribs, then all the way up to the top of your lungs, into your chest and up to your collarbones and heart. The breath will fill up your lungs from the bottom to the top, like the way a pitcher of water is filled.

When you empty your lungs, the breath will leave from the top (chest) to the middle (ribs) and lastly through the belly. You will feel your belly gently contract at the bottom of the exhale as you squeeze the last few drops of air out.

In the beginning, you may want to practice just 3-10 breath cycles. In that short amount of time, you will feel calmer and more relaxed and centered. As you practice, you can build to 2-5 minutes. Set a timer if that helps you.

4) Alternate Nostril Breath

This breathing exercise may seem a little weird for those who are new to a breathing practice, but it has a very calming and balancing effect on the mind and central nervous system, so it's worth a try.

Traditionally, this exercise is practiced seated, using your fingers to block the flow of breath through alternating nostrils. You can also practice on your back without using your fingers and instead just use your mind to imagine the breath coming in and out of alternating nostrils. I learned the second technique at a Yoga Therapy/ Yoga for Veterans training, as a way to help veterans heal from PTSD (Post Traumatic Stress Disorder). Follow these steps:

1) To begin, take the thumb of your right hand over your right nostril. Then take the middle and ring finger of your right hand over the left nostril.
2) Next, without closing either nostril, take a full breath cycle in through both nostrils.
3) Then, close off the right nostril with your right thumb and exhale through the left nostril.
4) Once you have exhaled completely through the left nostril, inhale through that same nostril.

5) Then, shift the pressure to close off the left nostril and exhale completely through the right nostril.
6) Then, inhale completely through the right nostril. At the top of the inhale, shift the pressure to close off the right nostril, exhaling through the left nostril.
7) Keep alternating and repeating for approximately 3-5 minutes or 5-10 breath cycles.

If you want to practice in corpse pose without using your fingers to block the flow of air, close your eyes and repeat the same sequence as above, simply imagining the airflow coming in and out of the alternating nostrils. This breathing technique takes practice but will have a very balancing effect on both hemispheres of the brain and the central nervous system.

Mindfulness, Meditation and Prayer

I decided to combine mindfulness, meditation and prayer because, even though they are all very different, I feel like the common thread is connecting to our higher power, single-tasking our mind and practicing our gratitude.

"If you are depressed you are living in the past. If you are anxious you are living in the future. If you are at peace you are living in the present."

– Lao Tzu

I was raised Catholic and grew up very comfortable with prayer. No matter your religion or beliefs, there is something so joyful and uplifting about feeling deep faith and a connection to God or a higher power. Being spiritual doesn't need to only happen with a formal religion or in a church. You can feel that connection while hiking a mountain, playing a sport, or being with someone you love.

I was first exposed to mindfulness training in the 90s

72

when I worked at Canyon Ranch Resort Spa in Lenox, Massachusetts. After taking a yoga class that taught breathing and mindfulness-based stress reduction, I bought Jon Kabat-Zinn's book *Wherever You Go There You Are.* Although it was first written almost 20 years ago (revised editions are now available), the message of single-tasking and being present is timeless.

Meditation is my favorite centering technique because it combines elements of both prayer and mindfulness. The misconception is that meditation is clearing and emptying your mind. In reality, it's more about finding peace and stillness and listening to your thoughts. We are so bombarded by music, advertisements screaming at us, incessant phone chatting all around us and constant noise pollution. It's hard to find quiet, so it's challenging to connect and listen to our thoughts. I crave silence so much, I often turn the radio off when driving.

While I was recovering from Lyme, I came across a guided imagery audio CD from Belleruth Naperstek that I used while doing acupuncture and meditation. The positive affirmations and visualizations were very powerful, putting me in a deep place of relaxation to reprogram my brain and to better handle the stress of chronic disease.

At one of my yoga trainings, my teacher read the ancient scripture called *The Musk Deer.* It was an ah-ha moment for me. The story is about a deer who spends his entire life running around looking for the answers to happiness. Like many of us, the deer looked in books, sought out gurus, asking everyone he knew for "the secret" to fulfillment.

At the end of his life, when the deer was dying, he finally found stillness. It was then that he smelled the musk scent he had frantically searched for his whole life. On the day of his birth, the scent was placed on his forehead, between his eyebrows (at his third eye chakra, which is the home of intuition and inner wisdom). His whole life, it had always been there. All he had to do was slow down and be still to find it. The moral of the story is that the answers are not found outside of us, but rather within us. To me, this is the goal of meditation.

Many athletes from championship winning NFL teams, NBA players, college athletes and Olympians have incorporated both yoga and mindfulness meditation into their sports training. Even Marines, CEOs and stressed out college students are learning to meditate for enhanced focus, improved memory and stress management. The way we train our brains is as important as how we train our bodies.

> *"As a Marine, the tools offered by consistent yoga and mindfulness practice allows me to see the full impact of traumatic combat experiences. Empowered with the insight to grow and evolve, I am stronger and more resilient than ever. It has brought harmony and ease to my mind and body. Yoga brought me home and saved my life."*
>
> **- CJ Keller, former Marine Corps Captain, OIF (Operation Iraqi Freedom) Veteran and yoga director for Warrior Wellness Solutions**

Meditation, prayer and mindfulness are opportunities to turn off the phone, the computer and the TV and simply let the mind and the body rest. It's a chance to unplug, surrender, heal, recover and be at peace. Ideally during a meditation, you stay fully awake and aware, but don't feel guilty if you fall asleep. Beyond breathing practice or meditation, the bigger picture is to train your mind and to be able to call upon that peace in challenging moments when you need it most.

In the beginning of a meditation practice, consider setting a timer for 3-5 minutes so you won't have to waste any of your focus on wondering how much time has passed (which is totally normal and does not mean you are doing it wrong). As you practice, you'll get more relaxed and comfortable and better able to focus your mind on your breathing and the present moment.

Consider practicing with a guided meditation, in silence, or to relaxing music. You will need to experiment to find out what works for you. There are many great free and paid meditation apps you can download too.

In yoga, we finish each class with final relaxation, otherwise known as Savasana (the pose of stillness). This brief time at the end of class allows you to be still and breathe, letting the work you did during class settle into every cell of your body and allowing the mind to relax as well.

For some, Savasana is their favorite pose that they look forward to all class. For others, stillness is torture and their mind races around to the past or into the future and their to-do list. Sometimes the thing we need the most is also the most challenging. If we only do what we're good at, life can get very unbalanced.

The power of prayer, mindfulness and meditation should not be minimized. Like anything worthwhile, it takes time, patience and practice to achieve the desired goal. I wonder what would happen if doctors prescribed meditation and prayer as often as they prescribe pills?

Tapping / EFT (Emotional Freedom Technique)

Tapping is a type of energy work that has an effect both on the meridians (energy lines) in the body as well as the psychology of the mind. It can help with everything from pre-race jitters and stress to chronic pain and childhood traumas.

I was first exposed to EFT through the Tapping World Summit, led by siblings Nick and Jessica Ortner. I'll admit I thought it was a little weird at first, tapping different points on my face and body while talking through a series of statements and affirmations.

EFT is based on the same energy meridians as traditional acupuncture points but without the needles. You tap on the energy points with your fingers while repeating affirmation type statements to clear and balance the mind and body.

Many people are skeptical of how powerful this simple and inexpensive (free unless you hire an EFT coach) tool can be. But after I participated in the Tapping World Summit for the past two years, I am a believer. Like yoga, meditation, or breathing exercises, it takes discipline to carve out time to practice EFT, but the results can be astounding. In the scheme of things, the time commitment is short since you can feel better in minutes.

One of my first experiences with EFT happened when I woke up with a migraine, ironically during the week of the Tapping World Summit. After Tapping along to a guided session (that just happened to be on the subject of pain that day), I drank a big glass of water with magnesium and took a nap. I woke up an hour later completely pain-free. Normally, when a migraine comes, I'd be in bed all day in agony. Instead I was able to go about my work day as planned.

If EFT is of interest to you I'd highly recommend participating in the free online event called the Tapping World Summit.

Essential Oils

People have been using essential oils for thousands of years for their natural healing qualities. I use them in the morning to wake up and before bed to help induce deeper sleep but you can use them anytime to lift mood, increase strength, induce healing and boost endurance. Calming oils are great to use with meditation and breathing practices to feel more centered and connected.

I've used essential oils for years in my yoga classes to help students feel more energized, balanced or relaxed. I sometimes use peppermint, tangerine or grapefruit oil on a grey, rainy day to uplift and energize the group. I typically use a lavender blend for final relaxation to help induce a calm sense of peace. Recently I began to better understand that essential oils are more than simply energizing or calming.

You can experiment with uplifting and energizing oils like peppermint, tangerine, grapefruit, rosemary, lemon and ginger; or calming oils like lavender and chamomile. Some pain-relieving oils include frankincense, which has anti-inflammatory properties, balsam fir and wintergreen, which have a similar feel to Icy Hot. Before a training session you could even try an oil that enhances strength and endurance like cedarwood, sandalwood, or rosemary.

Many essential oil companies combine several oils to create blends that can awaken the senses and create the desired effect. Many health food stores have demo samples you can experiment with to see what fragrances appeal to you. Intuitively, our senses guide us to make the best choice for what we need. If it smells good to you, go with it! Be aware, that like supplements, there are different ranges in quality for essential oils. Some are pure, natural, organic and very high quality while others are synthetic. It's worth spending a few extra dollars for quality.

Rescue a Dog

My favorite chillpower secret is my rescue pup Stella. No herbal concoction or breathing practice can get me more relaxed, happy and in the moment than my four legged furry friend.

The most important element of chillpower is being in the present moment, not stressing over the past or worrying about the future. That unconditional love and in-the-moment quality is a dog's greatest gift and it is infectious and contagious.

Stella is also a great workout partner. Studies show that dog owners have lower blood pressure and better overall health, so giving a rescue pup a second chance is absolutely a win-win. Technically, my husband and I rescued her, but Stella's enthusiastic, joyful spirit uplifts us both every day. We often wonder, who saved who?! While we were searching on Petfinder, my husband would say, "one of these dogs is going to win the lottery." But we both agree that we were the lottery winners. Rescuing a dog is priceless.

I know from other dog-loving owners that Stella is among many unofficial "therapy dogs" that bring joy unlike anything you can get in a bottle. I found Stella through Bonnie Blue Rescue and there are thousands of animals in shelters all across the country and on Petfinder.com. Dogs are not for everyone. Like any relationship, it's a commitment and it requires work and some sacrifice. But, to me, the rewards far outweigh the investment and unlike blood pressure drugs or antidepressants, the only side effect you'll feel is joy!

Strengthen Your Shield

Strengthening your protective shield means boosting your immune system and protecting your health and body. A warrior can often miss this key element. Entering a battle, work day or game day at less than 100 percent puts you at greater risk for injury, not being mentally or physically sharp and regretting not doing your best.

Sacrificing your peace and recovery isn't doing anyone any good. An injured, burned out warrior can't go into battle as their highest self. No matter if your battle is a day at the office, managing your kids' schedules and meals, or heading into a championship game, learning how to harness the power of rest, recovery and re-fueling is the secret to achieving new levels of greatness.

One of the many things I love about yoga is that you challenge, stretch and strengthen your body, followed by stillness and relaxation. I have had students that actually hate Savasana and find it miserable to be still and relax. I have had students that love stillness and only come to class for the Savasana. Which kind of student are you?

No matter your feelings on Savasana, the reality is that the only time your body repairs and grows stronger is while it is at rest. If you live by the quote "You can rest when you're dead" you might be at risk of not being your best while you're alive. If you think that being still isn't a productive use of your time, you couldn't be more wrong. I'm certainly not encouraging you to be a couch potato and watch more TV. We're talking about quality rest, which is one of the most beneficial immune system strengtheners.

When your immune system is balanced and strong, you are more resistant to getting sick and are also less likely to get an autoimmune disease. An anti-inflammatory diet will improve your immune function, helping you to fight disease and common infections while reducing inflammation.

I think it's better to prevent a battle, but if you need to fight, you want to be your strongest. Sometimes, like in sports, we know when those physical challenges are coming and we can be prepared. Other times we get blindsided with an infection, injury or even an accident. Keep your armor and shield strong every day and your internal warriors ready to fight at any given moment, so they are there for you when you need them most. If you do get sick, take time for self-care. The world won't end if you take a day off and your office mates will be grateful you didn't spread your germs.

Toxic Toiletries

Your skin is an important part of your protective shield. Think of it as your armor and your first line of defense. What we put on our skin is absorbed into our body. In addition to choosing cleaner, unprocessed organic foods when possible, choosing organic skin care and non-toxic home cleaners can help to limit your exposure to chemicals, which can weaken your protective shield over time and lead to generalized unwellness. Read labels. You might be surprised at the amount of chemicals in many products, such as:

- Skin care, toiletries, toothpaste, deodorants, soaps, makeup, lotions and perfumes
- Home cleaners, candles, detergents and scented room fragrances
- Environmental pollutants like lawn and garden chemicals

As you clean up your diet and clean out your kitchen pantry and refrigerator, consider detoxifying your home and make up bag. You may be inspired to do a full home and body detox to clean the slate and start fresh. Or you may take it slow and simply replace items little by little. Either way, know that what you put on your skin and what you breathe can affect your health. As a side note, I believe toxic relationships can make you physically sick and either weaken or strengthen you in every way, so choose the people you surround yourself with wisely.

My favorite resources for toxin-free living include Kris Carr, FOODMATTERS, Josh Axe and Wellness Mama. Do your research and dump the toxins.

Colonic/Colon Hydrotherapy

It is said that all disease starts in the colon and that approximately 70 percent of your immune function lies in your digestive tract. It's not just what we're eating that affects our health, it's what we're absorbing! If your colon is jammed up due to an unhealthy diet, dehydration, illness and medications, your immune system might not be functioning at its peak.

You could be eating a super healthy diet and spending lots of money on supplements, but not absorbing all their benefits. That money and those good intentions are then literally flushed down the toilet! In addition, health issues that we don't associate with our colon (like susceptibility to colds and flu, headaches, acne, hormonal problems and fatigue) can often trace back to the digestive tract.

While I believe our bodies are equipped to naturally take care of most things, we now live in an environment where we are exposed to so many unnatural foods, medications and environmental toxins that our bodies weren't created to handle.

A colonic is an alternative medical therapy that cleanses the colon and intestinal tract, flushing out accumulated waste. While there is no scientific evidence of the benefits of colon hydrotherapy, there have been times where I went in for a colonic with a headache or backache and left without one. Since a colonic flushes your colon with water, it is very hydrating. Many pains, including headaches, are due to simple dehydration so it's possible the hydrating effect is what cured my pain.

I'm not a big fan of anything that interferes with mother nature. Having said that, I do feel like colonics have helped me with the side effects of a 7 months of antibiotics for Lyme. Had I known about probiotics and a proper diet at the time of my treatment, my colon may not have gotten in such bad shape. Maybe my colon is better able to absorb nutrients now that it's cleaner. Or maybe it's my imagination. Either way, I don't get sick as often as I used to and my headaches, acne and muscle pain have decreased significantly.

The less toxic our lifestyle, the less we need something like a colonic. In a world that is now filled with chemicals and man-made GMOs (genetically modified organisms), cheese curls and diet soda, I feel my digestive tract has benefitted from an occasional colonic spring cleaning. However, if you don't have any health issues, are a lifelong healthy eater and have regular bowel movements, you probably could do without a colonic.

As with all self-care, talk to your doctor first and ask your friends and family for referrals. Don't schedule a colonic unless you've gotten a good referral from a trusted source.

Probiotics

Probiotics are good bacteria and microorganisms that can improve health and digestion as well as immune function. The combination of antibiotics, depleted soil and an ultra-clean freak mentality (where we douse our hands with antibacterial soaps and lotions constantly) has been causing us lots of problems and killing off good bacteria with the bad.

If you're eating locally grown fruits and vegetables from a CSA (Community Supported Agriculture) farm or farmers market, you never take antibiotics and don't use antibacterial products, you might not need to supplement with probiotics. Most of us are not exposed to enough of these healthy "good guy" bacteria and could use a supplemental boost.

Cultured and fermented foods like yogurt, kefir, sauerkraut and kombucha drinks are also great ways to increase the good bacteria in your gut and boost your immune system. For supplements, I switch around to different brands frequently to increase exposure to a variety of good bacteria strains. I also make a habit of taking probiotics before, during and after travel. I've even made my own kombucha and sauerkraut, but this takes time and a bit of practice. With convenient products like kefir and KeVita brand probiotic drinks now widely available, it is easy to keep your good-guy warrior cells outnumbering and stronger than the bad guys!

Stress

Your diet and exercise regime could be perfect, but if your marriage is a wreck and your finances are upside down then stress can cause havoc with your health despite your being physically fit. Factor relationships, joy and stress management into your self-care equation.

Have you ever had a bad dream and woke up sweaty with your heart pounding? You were safe in your bed the entire time, but what went on in your head transported you to a place of fear and anxiety. The same goes with watching a scary movie. You know you are safe, but your heart still races with fear. Think back to a time when you were very stressed and how it affected your sleep and every aspect of your life.

Everyone responds differently to stress and so much of that reaction is in our head. Just like how our body responds to a bad dream, what goes on in our mind affects our blood pressure, heart rate, hormones, sleep, what we eat, how we store fat and even our emotions.

The fight-or-flight response is there to protect us from danger, but in our current society, stress has become constant instead of an occasional threat. This state of chronic stress affects our body and health in endless ways. Fortunately we can manage our stress with simple tools like breathing, exercise, meditation and the choices we make. A less-is-more approach to life and exercise can reduce stress, lower cortisol levels and provide a sense of peace that calms and strengthens your immune system.

Adrenal fatigue is also a serious issue for thousands of people who constantly push themselves to the limit. Overtraining and over-exercising often backfires because it puts our body into a self-induced stress and survival "fight or flight" mode which raises cortisol levels and depletes our adrenals. Many folks resort to using sleep aids and alcohol to help them deal with stress or sleep better and then stimulants like caffeine and sugar to pick their energy up again. This only further complicates matters and throws us further off balance.

I hope the pendulum will start to swing back to a place where it's more fashionable to be relaxed, patient and stress-free than to be frazzled, rushed and tense. Our immune systems, health and happiness will all benefit from a less-is-more approach.

My good friend Ian Wasti wrote a short, lighthearted book called, *The Perfect Antidote - Why Greatness is Overrated*. His refreshing approach to get back to basics encourages us to sometimes lower the bar, procrastinate or "get a smaller plate" in order to create a new perspective and experience more happiness.

For many high achievers, it may sound counter-intuitive to lower your expectations. While Ian's message is not about reducing stress, part of the underlying theme is to stress less and enjoy more. By no means is it a message to give up and never set goals. To me, his message is about experiencing more peace in your life by finding the balance between "never give up" and "always let go."

All the self-care in the world won't help if you're continually stressing your mind and body. It's like changing your tires but your alignment is off or patching the ceiling but not fixing the leaky roof. The Band-Aid approach may temporarily cover up the problem and mask symptoms but getting to the source of your stress is the best long-term self-care solution.

It's counterproductive to get stressed about creating your self-care plan. Be flexible and relaxed in your approach. The foods we eat and stretches we do are only part of the equation. How we feel when we are eating and stretching matters just as much if not more. A more healthy, flexible mind and body comes with calmness, quality sleep and a resilient response to stress.

"Be gentle with yourself.
You are a child of the universe,
no less than the trees and the stars.
In the noisy confusion of life,
keep peace in your soul."

– Max Ehrmann

"Flexibility means being able to make problems into teachers."

– Dadi Janki

"The hard and still will be broken. The soft and supple will prevail."

– Lao Tzu

"Notice that the stiffest tree is easily cracked while the bamboo survives by bending with the wind."

– Eleanor Brownn

4

Flexibility for Warriors

> *"Everybody is a genius. But if you judge a fish by its ability to climb a tree, it will live its whole life believing that it is stupid."*
>
> **– Albert Einstein**

For many strong warrior types, flexibility is not our greatest strength. If this is true for you, the first thing you should do is accept your flexibility as it is right now. Too often people won't practice what they're not good at, which only creates more imbalance. Avoid judging your flexibility. There is no such thing as being bad at yoga.

Keep in mind that being too flexible, physically or mentally, can also get you in trouble. Over-stretching and hypermobility can lead to joint instability and injury. Being too mentally flexible can lead to being a doormat and never doing what you want when you want. Strive for a healthy sense of flexibility balanced with strength.

What does flexibility have to do with power? The most powerful athletes are strong, fast and flexible. Range of motion directly affects an athlete's physical power. Think of a rubber band, a bow and arrow or when a golfer winds up to tee off. How far an object propels forward is directly related to how far it can draw back. Limited range of motion limits power but it also increases your chances of injury. When a body is stiff and lacks mobility, it's more likely to get strained. You want to bend without breaking.

Before we talk specifically about stretching, also consider how flexible you are within your strength and cardio routine. We are creatures of habit and can tend to get stuck in a rut instead of cross training and finding variety. Adding more whole body, functional training that includes flexibility exercises will reduce overuse injuries, so mix it up and try new things.

There is a lot of confusing and conflicting information about stretching. Some think stretching is a waste of time or can even hurt performance. Others feel it's indispensable for peak performance. The topic of stretching is very much like the world of nutrition where so many diets and contradictory information make it hard to know what to eat.

Effective recovery isn't as simple as sitting on the couch. Your recovery will vary depending on your training and body, but active recovery means you participate in some sort of cross training activity, like yoga, foam rolling or Pilates. A coach or trainer can help you choose the best recovery technique to suit your goals and training schedule as well as budget your time to include flexibility training. It's our job as coaches to know when to push for more and when to ask for less, so that our clients know and understand the importance of balance and flexibility and never leave a session feeling frazzled and tight.

I've experimented a lot with flexibility training and have come to the conclusion that different styles of stretching work best for different people. We are all very unique so finding the style of stretching that works for you is much like a childhood fairy tale *Goldilocks and The Three Bears*.

What Does Goldilocks Have To Do With Flexibility?

When people are new to yoga and stretching, I advise them to try a variety of class styles and teachers until they find the one that clicks with them. Some classes may be too hot or fast-paced while others may be too cold or slow-paced. Some teachers may be too weird for you and others may not be relaxing or spiritual enough for your taste.

Finding the class that is "just right" is a bit like Goldilocks finding the perfect porridge. It's worth the effort to find a class and teacher that suits your preferences, goals and personality. If you don't find the right match on your first try, try again! There are also many DVDs and online classes available for you to practice with in your own home. Or you can hire a private teacher so the training is customized just for you. The options are limitless.

If you're an athlete, practice a more gentle, restorative yoga during your in-season and incorporate cross training with a more athletic style in the off-season. If you are new to yoga, don't let all the different style choices intimidate you. Start with a beginner level class to build a strong foundation before moving on to an intermediate or advanced level class.

I've summarized the most common styles of yoga, stretching and mind-body exercises for reference, but know that classes will vary depending on the teacher and studio, so ask before you enter a class. There are a huge variety of mind-body classes now available and many combine elements of many different styles. There are yoga boot camps, Pilates-yoga fusion classes and even Spinning and yoga combo classes. Experiment to find what suits your goals and taste.

Hatha Yoga is the umbrella term which all other styles fall under. "Ha" means "sun" and "tha" means "moon" so it's really about the balance of opposites. Typically Hatha classes are very traditional and fairly gentle in nature. Hatha refers to the physical yoga practice but if you see "Hatha" on the schedule it is often a moderately-paced, all-level class with basic poses and breathing exercises.

Vinyasa/Flow/Ashtanga or Power Yoga all refer to a movement based often athletic and active class formats that incorporate Sun Salutations, a series of twelve poses linked together to energize and warm the body. The pace and degree of difficulty can vary significantly depending on the teacher and studio, but for the most part be prepared for a challenging total body workout. There are also "hot vinyasa" style classes in a heated room, which increase the sweat factor even more.

Yin/Restorative classes are focused on more gentle, relaxing poses at a slow and easy pace for recovery, stress management and relaxation. Often there will be props used such as bolsters, blankets and straps for supported poses. Yin is quiet and meditative while yang refers to the more active, movement-based styles of yoga, like vinyasa flow.

Iyengar/Anusara are both styles that focus more on proper alignment and longer holds. Although alignment is important in all styles of yoga, it is taken more seriously in

Iyengar, which uses many props to get you into perfect alignment in all poses. Anusara is a more lighthearted, less strict version of Iyengar that uses fewer props. If you love perfection and alignment, then Iyengar may be a fit for you.

Hot Yoga/Bikram Yoga are both taught in high heat, but they are very different in style. Bikram yoga classes are typically 90 minutes long and are in a 104 degree room. The format is 60 poses done in the same order every class. If you like high heat and repetition, then try Bikram. Hot yoga or hot vinyasa classes are usually in an 80-95 degree room and the pose sequences vary depending on the class and instructor. So if you want more variety with your high heat yoga, try hot yoga or hot vinyasa.

Many athletic types are drawn to Bikram or hot yoga classes because of the intense heat and killer sweat. Be aware there are advantages and disadvantages to hot yoga. Studies show that practicing yoga in the high heat can help athletes endure heat for their sport and improve range of motion. The concern is that athletes can tend to be competitive and be more prone to over stretch in high heat. In addition, dehydration can be an issue, so drink a lot of water.

For the non-athlete, there is a perceived exertion factor to consider too. Standing still in a 110 degree room could still produce a lot of sweat. Keep in mind that sweating buckets doesn't necessarily mean you worked that hard. Be realistic about your effort.

Tai Chi and Qigong are both gentle and good for all levels. Both disciplines originated in China and involve slow, gentle movements that help to improve energy and balance and reduce stress. Neither discipline is focused on a lot of stretching or flexibility, but can improve balance and range of motion and increase energy and mindfulness while creating a calming effect on the central nervous system.

Pilates is very different from yoga but some of the

benefits are similar. Pilates is excellent for core strength, balance and flexibility. It incorporates repetitions of callisthenic-type exercises that improve total body endurance and strength with a focus on the core. Pilates can help to reduce back pain and improve posture. As with yoga, there are many different styles and levels of Pilates, so if you're just beginning, try an entry-level class.

Ki-Hara is a dynamic style of flexibility that both strengthens and stretches the entire body while engaging the core. Resistance is used during the stretches to engage the muscles both concentrically and eccentrically, so there is strength within your range of motion. Keeping the muscle engaged throughout the movement allows for greater power and stability and prevents overstretching. Ki-Hara offers self-stretches, where you provide your own resistance, and assisted stretches, where a trainer provides the resistance for the stretches. Ki-Hara also includes mashing, a style of bodywork that helps loosen-up and prepare muscles for stretching and helps flush and release toxins after stretching.

Athletic/Sports Stretching is typically an old school approach to flexibility that coaches and personal trainers use to stretch out all major muscle groups. A few minutes of basic athletic stretches after a workout can reduce stiffness, increase range of motion and improve recovery. Stretching doesn't need to be fancy or take an hour at a yoga studio. Your stretch routine can be as simple as 5-10 minutes of basic stretching.

Although many people skip stretching, flexibility is one of the three basic elements of fitness, along with strength and cardiovascular endurance. The key with all these styles of stretching is experimenting with

"The journey of a thousand miles begins with a single step."

– Lao Tzu

an open mind, especially in the beginning. Consistency and patience is essential. Start slowly, progress and build gradually. Begin your journey and keep putting one foot in front of the other.

The Difference Between Static & Dynamic Stretching

When most people think of stretching, they visualize static stretching, which involves holding a lengthened position for 30-60 seconds. Static stretches are less active and are more relaxing in nature. As you hold a static stretch and breathe, you allow the muscle to lengthen on its own. Studies on static stretching have found that it has a positive effect when done after a run or workout, but can decrease power or speed if done before a run or workout. Save your static stretching for your cool-down.

Static stretching can be done with or without a stretch strap, a simple tool to assist you in your stretches. You can use an old belt or tie or purchase a stretch band or yoga strap. My favorite is the Stretch Out Strap from OPTP.

Dynamic stretching is movement based and repetitive in nature. The goal with dynamic stretching is to move in and out of stretches smoothly and rhythmically to increase range of motion as you go. The yoga Sun Salutation is an example of an energizing, dynamic series of poses that take the body through full range of motion. It's the perfect warm up before a run or to do first thing in the morning to wake up.

When and how you stretch is important. Static stretching is better after a workout as part of your cool-down and dynamic stretching is preferred before a workout as part of your warm-up. Talk to your trainer to help you set up a flexibility program.

The concept behind "Flexible Warrior" is the balance of opposites: stability with mobility, strength with flexibility, calmness with energy, and humility with power. You can apply these principles to your yoga practice and to your life.

It's important to set an intention and know what you want and how you want to feel. Breathe deeply and fully. Align your body as well as your thoughts and your actions. Have integrity. Be balanced. Connect with the present moment. Do your best, but don't push over your edge. Practice with dedication but know when to let go.

1) Intention. As soon as you step onto your yoga mat, you are in a training session. Take a seated or standing mountain pose with your hands at heart center in prayer and set an intention. Dedicate your practice to someone or something greater than yourself. Why are you practicing? What do you want to get out of the session? How do you want to feel?

   Tip - Add "yoga" to your calendar. Write down your intentions and keep them posted with your training schedule.

2) Breathe. The most powerful tool to relax and focus your mind is breathing. Creating a calm energy with your breath can reduce anxiety and help keep you focused during distractions and challenging moments. Inhale deeply, filling your lungs and exhale completely, emptying your lungs. Pause and repeat.

3) Align, balance and connect. A strong core and an

aligned, balanced body is open, relaxed, strong and resilient. Stack and align your joints. Lift and open your heart. Stand tall. Create a connection to your core and to the present moment. It's not about touching our toes. It's about functional flexibility, range of motion and power with peace.

4) Find the edge. The edge is the fine line between pushing too hard and taking it too easy. You want to function at the top of your ability to maximize form and performance, but be able to stay relaxed. Pace yourself. Resist the temptation to push beyond your limit where you sacrifice form or expose yourself to injury. An over-trained warrior has less of a chance to win the battle. You're not doing yourself or your team any favors when you're hurt or exhausted. Always do your best, but be smart and protect yourself so you can continue to move forward and fight.

5) Practice and rest. Discipline and consistency will get you results, but so will rest and recovery. Know when to push and when to surrender.

The three most important things to remember when stretching are:

1) Don't overstretch or strain. If you're shaking or holding your breath you are overstretching. Less is more when stretching. Consistency is what will get you results, not forcing.

2) Breathe. Most importantly, don't hold your breath!

3) Hit all the major muscle groups, not just the ones that are feeling tight. Often, the opposing muscle group is the cause or a contributing factor to tightness.

Don't get too caught up in all the rules and doing the poses exactly right. While form, safety and alignment are important, what's more important is how you feel. The number one rule is, if it feels good, you're doing it right. If it hurts or you're holding your breath, something needs to change.

Like nutrition, training and even running shoes, everyone responds differently and not one size fits all. Approach your flexibility training with a sense of flexibility. If you approach your stretching with a strict, rigid, closed mind, your body will react, so relax. Chillpower!

Make sure when you're taking a yoga class that you are mindful of your alignment and that you listen to the messages your body is sending instead of forcing and competing.

Stretching Basics:

- Hold each static stretch for about 5 breath cycles or 30 seconds.
- Repeat static stretches 2-6 times.
- Stretch 3-4 times a week at minimum, but 5-7 days is ideal. This can be a combination of both static and dynamic stretching.
- Stretching for just 10 minutes a day can be very effective, so make that your minimum goal.
- Vary your flexibility methods to see what feels and works best for your body. Experiment with static, dynamic and Ki-Hara techniques.
- Try using heating pads and foam rolling before and after stretching to see if it helps increase your range of motion and decrease soreness.
- Consider working with a personal trainer or one-on-one stretch trainer.

- Stretch all major muscle groups and remember the opposing muscle groups.
- Find the edge in each stretch. Stretch to your limit but not to the point of shaking or pain.
- Breathe slowly, fully and deeply while stretching.
- Vary the stretches slightly to target different areas of tension.
- Stretch after each workout and focus on relaxing the mind and body.

When you don't have time to make it to a class, there are plenty of stretch sequences you can do at home. If you are better at following along as a teacher talks you through, there are many free segments available on Youtube. You can check out my Flexible Warrior channel: (www.youtube.com/flexiblewarrioryoga) or search for other teachers and formats that suit your taste.

Self-Massage

Getting massage regularly can be expensive, so self-massage is a great and inexpensive way to keep the benefits of your massage lasting longer. Taking extra time to work on the spots that need extra attention can have huge benefits.

Self-myofascial release (SMR) can break up areas of tension, especially when done regularly after your workouts and before you sleep. You can use a foam roller or other tools like The Stick or Yoga Tune Up Balls. I like wearing compression gear when foam rolling so clothes don't bunch up and get in the way of deep tissue work.

Trigger points are painful knots in the tissue that are often sore and inflamed. You want to approach these sore spots with caution, giving enough pressure to increase blood flow and relax the tissue, but not so much that it increases inflammation and creates further trauma. When you find a trigger point during a self-massage session, spend extra time on that spot. Take a few deep breaths while you massage that spot and release the soreness.

My favorite references for self-massage are Jill Miller's Yoga Tune Up, Sue Hitzmann's The Melt Method and Kelly Starrett's MobilityWOD. Great self-myofascial release tools are available at TriggerPoint, Rumble Roller and OPTP. My Flexible Warrior Foam Roll & Stretch DVD is available at www.spinervals.com

Run with a High Heart

Stretching and posture are boring topics for many. I often wonder how we can make stretching sexier and more exciting, but the truth is the motivation is in the results. Slouching is not sexy.

Overtraining often creates imbalance which can create bad posture and injuries. I've been there, hobbling around with a tweaked knee, achy back or barely able to turn my head due to a strained neck. It can make you feel old, depressed and grouchy.

Aligned posture and pain-free running feels great and has a positive effect on your outlook, too. Try it for a second. Go ahead and slouch. When your shoulders round forward, your head drops, your spine slumps and you look and feel defeated. Slouching closes off your heart and chest and restricts your breathing. When you sit or stand tall, lifting your heart and bringing your spine into alignment, you can breathe more freely and will feel and look more empowered and proud. Good posture is definitely more attractive plus it improves performance. Pilates and yoga are both great to build core strength and better alignment.

I realize I'm a geek, but I watch people's form and posture when they are playing sports and running. Many athletes have a rounded posture. In the fitness world, we call this kyphosis. This hunchback posture is chronic in our culture due to the activities of daily living including sitting, typing, driving and walking with our faces in our phones. Even gardening and cooking can put our spine into flexion, rounding our posture.

Running for miles after sitting all day further exacerbates the issue. The next thing you know, you're in a chronic state of slump and your neck and back hurt. Then you take drugs to dull that pain when all you really need is to strengthen your back and align your posture. Performance, body composition and physique all improve when you cross train and have a strong core, a balanced body and good posture.

You may hear the phrase "lead with your heart" in yoga class. This term is not just referring to heart-centered leadership skills and work ethic. It's also about movement patterns. Leading with your heart and keeping your chest lifted immediately brings your posture into better alignment. When you apply this lifted posture to your running, it allows you to breathe better and use better body mechanics. Over time, this can make a big difference in injury prevention and performance.

Early in my running career, I invested in the book *ChiRunning: A Revolutionary Approach to Effortless, Injury-free Running*. I was intrigued with reducing injury and improving performance with simple principles and form adjustments. For anyone interested in running pain-free, I'd highly recommend checking out ChiRunning. My hope is to one day see everyone smiling as they run with a high heart.

Flexibility Within Flexibility

Just like styles of yoga, there are many different approaches to stretching. Within those variations are different personalities of stretching trainers. Since we're all so unique, it's impossible for me to write a program that specifically meets your individual flexibility needs. Find a personal trainer or stretch trainer in your area can who can customize a flexibility program specifically for you!

"The food you eat can either be the safest and most powerful form of medicine or the slowest form of poison."

– Ann Wigmore

"The doctor of the future will no longer treat the human frame with drugs, but rather will cure and prevent disease with nutrition."

– Thomas Edison

"We pay the doctor to make us better when we really should be paying the farmer to keep us healthy."

– Robyn O'Brien

5

Eat for Flexibility

What you eat affects your body in every way, including your flexibility. How you eat is as important as what you eat. Approaching your diet with a flexible, open mind instead of being rigid will bring you more variety, joy, freedom and health. You don't necessarily need to count calories, carbs or grams of sugar if you eat mostly non-processed, real foods and less fake, manufactured "frankenfoods."

My diet changes day by day, month by month and year by year. No matter what dietary approach I follow on any given day, minimizing processed foods and increasing a variety of natural whole foods reduces inflammation, prevents disease and increases strength, energy and vitality. When the body has less inflammation, it is more resilient and able to move and stretch freely.

I was introduced to Bio-individuality™ as a student at the Integrative Institute of Nutrition (IIN)®. This dietary theory is all about flexibility and reinforces the importance of listening to our body, trusting our intuition and acknowledging that we each have different chemistry. In addition, our dietary needs may change at different phases of our life. What works for me may not work for you.

While I worked at Canyon Ranch Resort Spa, I had the opportunity to take a workshop with nutritional psychologist Marc David, who published a book called *Nourishing Wisdom*. His workshop introduced me to the concept that how we eat is as important as what we eat. Our thoughts, mood and attitude toward food as well as what we do while we eat can affect how we assimilate nutrients. Mindlessly eating healthy food when you're rushing, angry or stressed is counterproductive. The more stressed and uptight you are, the less resilient and flexible you will be. This concept includes your approach to diet, too.

Instead of strict rules that exclude food groups and overwhelm you with complicated guidelines and recipes, you'll have the flexibility to choose wisely with no guilt. You will increase your consumption of healthy, anti-inflammatory foods and decrease processed, inflammatory junk foods. The IIN term for this concept is "crowding out," which basically means that the more healthy food you eat, the less room there is for junk food.

There are hundreds of diets on the market that you can experiment with, depending on your personal goals. My goal is to reduce inflammation and increase healing and energy. The five dietary approaches I have gotten the greatest benefit from are: anti-inflammatory, paleo, vegetarian, raw food and superfoods. All five of these diets provide anti-inflammatory healing benefits. Incorporating elements from all five plans offers great variety and unlimited options.

At first, I felt undisciplined with my all-over-the-board dietary approach. Then I found out it had a name: *flexitarian*. Since I'm all about flexibility, taking a flexitarian/omnivore approach is a perfect match.

The Flexitarian Diet was written by Dawn Jackson Blatner and is considered a semi-vegetarian approach, focusing on mostly plant-based foods and occasionally including animal proteins. When I read about this flexible approach I felt immediately aligned with the principles, which allow a wide variety of healthy choices without being overly restrictive.

An omnivore eats a variety of both plant and animal foods. With the abundance of food choices in our world today, being an omnivore is fun and slightly overwhelming. Michael Pollan's book *The Omnivore's Dilemma* offers great insight on the history and evolution of our food industry and how our choices affect our health, our planet and the future of both.

Diets for Healing and Recovery

No matter what dietary approach you choose, everyone can benefit from eating more vegetables, reducing foods that cause inflammation and increasing foods that promote healing. In addition to preventing disease, other great side effects of reduced inflammation are: increased energy and flexibility, improved recovery and mood and even weight loss and longevity.

> *"Eat food. Not too much. Mostly plants."*
>
> **- Michael Pollan, *In Defense of Food: An Eater's Manifesto***

The Anti-Inflammatory Diet is known to heal and prevent the chronic inflammation that causes most, if not all, diseases. I believe it also helps to reduce overall inflammation that can, over time, create the Tin Man effect, reducing range of motion, slowing recovery and restricting flexibility. Dr. Andrew Weil's anti-inflammatory approach is basically a Mediterranean diet with some added tweaks to make it even more effective. It's realistic and sustainable yet powerful and holistic.

Dr. Weil's Anti-Inflammatory Food Pyramid is balanced, easy to understand and user-friendly. It includes a lot of fruits and veggies, whole grains, beans and legumes, healthy fats like nuts, seeds and avocados, mushrooms, animal proteins and soy, eggs, yogurt, cheese, herbs and spices, tea, supplements, red wine and healthy sweets like dark chocolate. What you won't see on the anti-inflammatory diet are processed foods.

Dr. Josh Axe created a *Healing Foods Diet* that has anti-inflammatory qualities. The foods on his shopping list are high quality, nutrient-dense, real foods and his approach is practical and easy to follow. You'll stock up on veggies, wild caught fish, raw dairy, organic, grass-fed meats, nuts and seeds, high-quality oils, berries, spices, superfoods and herbs. You can download his shopping list and recipes for free! Creating vibrant health doesn't have to be complicated. Follow Dr. Axe on Facebook and Twitter for endless health and fitness inspiration.

Raw Foods and Superfoods were a totally new concept when my health coach, Kendell Reichhart, introduced it and invited me to a raw food cooking class she was teaching. I wondered why we needed a cooking class if it was all raw food. The concept sounded weird to me. After the class I had a much better understanding and I was soon making green smoothies, incorporating superfoods and eating a wide variety of salads, sprouts and fresh juices. I even invested in a juicer and a Vitamix to make fresh juices and smoothies.

The idea with eating raw food is that cooking kills a lot of the natural enzymes and lowers nutritional value. As a yogi, I'm all about prana (life force energy) so eating more foods that have their prana intact makes sense to me. I enjoyed these foods so much I took a weekend workshop with raw food expert David Avocado Wolfe which opened my eyes to a whole new world of healing superfoods and superherbs.

Superfoods are one of the easiest and most effective ways to boost energy, speed recovery and improve performance. Aside from providing fuel, superfoods provide essential nutrients, assist with repairing our muscles and connective tissue and help build muscle to keep us strong.

Eating seasonally and enjoying more raw foods in the spring and summer makes sense. When the weather is warm, we can get fresh local fruits and veggies from the CSA and the farmers market. Raw foods, superfoods and superherbs are an excellent addition to boost your diet. Look for recipe ideas from FOODMATTERS TV, Kris Carr and David Wolfe.

The Paleo Diet is known to be healing for people with inflammatory issues and autoimmune disease, so I was very motivated to try this diet. Paleo focuses on reducing inflammatory Omega-6 fatty acids found in processed junk foods and increasing healthy Omega-3s found in pastured eggs, wild-caught fish and grass-fed meats. Paleo foods include lean proteins, fruit, vegetables and healthy fats, like avocados, olive oil, nuts and seeds while avoiding dairy, grains, sugars and processed foods, all of which can cause inflammation and disease.

Since my blood type is O, the paleo diet was similar to the *The Blood Type Diet* that was recommended to me years ago when I was first diagnosed with thyroid disease. I bought *The Blood Type Diet* book but had a hard time sticking to the protocol since type O's are recommended to eat a lot of meat, which didn't appeal to me at the time. I wanted to be blood type A, which supposedly does better as a vegetarian; or blood type B, which does well with dairy; or the best of both worlds, blood type AB, which is believed to do well digesting dairy and being a vegetarian.

Even though I have "caveman blood," I rarely crave meat. I attribute this partly to my lifelong love of animals and more recently to my education in factory farming and animal cruelty. For great information, check resources from paleo experts like Robb Wolf, Chris Kesser and autoimmune thyroid specialists Izabella Wentz and Dr. Amy Myers. Like all dietary theories, there is conflicting information on protein consumption and whether or not animal protein is "acid-forming", which some believe causes inflammation and disease. You can make your own opinion on the acid-alkaline debate, based on how your body feels after you eat acidic foods like grains and meats.

More and more, there are local, organic farmers that offer free-range, grass-fed meats. The flexitarian approach allows us to dabble with both paleo and vegetarian recipes, which works well with the Flexible Warrior balance of opposites principle.

Vegetarians and vegans don't eat meat. Often vegetarians eat dairy and eggs, but vegans avoid all animal foods and products, like leather and wool. Plant-based diets are good for our planet because they reduce pollution and the depletion of our natural resources which come from the factory- farming of animals. A diet high in plant-foods reduces the risk of many diseases, but other benefits include weight loss, longevity, bone strength and increased energy.

A plant-based diet can be very healing and anti-inflammatory. Be aware that all processed foods can cause inflammation, even if they are vegan. Don't be a junk-food vegetarian. Also, any foods you are allergic or sensitive to can cause inflammation, vegetarian or not. Some studies conclude you will have less inflammation if you eat more vegetables and fruit, but many vegetarian diets are high in grains, which can cause inflammation when eaten in excess. Educate yourself and experiment.

Vegetarians and vegans are no longer just hippies or yogis. There are more and more plant-eating athletes, known as "*plantathletes*" who fuel their powerful and lean bodies on vegetables alone and avoid processed foods. For inspiration and recipes check out Brendan Brazier, Rich Roll and Matt Frazier, *the No Meat Athlete*. You can get a lot of great information on Twitter, Facebook, Instagram and Pinterest.

As a student at IIN, I was inspired by a speech by Venus Williams who switched to a plant-based diet to heal from Sjogren's syndrome. I also learned about Brendan Brazier's The *Thrive Diet*, a vegan approach that reduces inflammation by limiting stressful lifestyle and food choices. His focus is an anti-inflammatory diet full of fruits, vegetables and legumes. Also check out fitness expert Ben Greenfield's podcast for endless inspiration for athletic performance and everything from paleo to vegan.

If you need more motivation to add veggies into your diet, watch the documentary *Powered by Green Smoothies* by Sergei Boutenko. He tracked ten ultra-runners and CrossFitters who boosted their performance, reduced inflammation and improved recovery time by drinking a big green smoothie every day for six weeks.

Green smoothies and juices can be an acquired taste and results may vary from person to person, depending on food allergies, recipes and consistency of use. More and more, there are vegan and vegetarian athletes proving that you don't need to eat meat to perform at your peak. A flexitarian approach is semi-vegetarian which allows moderate portions of animal protein. Either way, eating a diet packed full of nutrient-dense vegetables and fruits is one of the most healing dietary changes you can make both for your body and the planet. Smoothies and fresh juices are one way to add more fruits and vegetables to your diet.

The Flexitarian Diet is mostly vegetarian, but doesn't eliminate meat completely. I love having the flexibility to cook a vegetarian dish for meatless Monday and a paleo recipe on Tuesday. This flexible approach keeps the choices unlimited, the variety huge and the balance in check. With so many diets on the market, it's hard to know which one to follow! But no one ever argues against the benefit of reducing junk food and adding more veggies to your diet.

Fuel Your Prana. Toss Your Kryptonite.

Prana is the life force energy that is inherent in all living things. Foods that strengthen your prana will reduce inflammation and your chances of disease. Foods that weaken your life force and increase inflammation are your kryptonite. To keep it simple, think energy = prana and garbage = kryptonite.

By limiting inflammatory kryptonite foods and increasing healing anti-inflammatory superfoods, you will fuel your prana and every cell in your body. If you are used to a disciplined, restricted diet, counting calories and carbs or feeling guilty about eating, the freedom of the Flexible Warrior approach might seem rebellious. For others, it will be exciting to focus simply on choosing foods that fuel your prana and limiting foods that drain or deplete you.

"It's not about the quantity of food or the calories, it's about the quality of food and its nutritional density."

-Kendell Reichhart, Holistic Health Coach

Keep in mind, it's not just the foods we eat that can either nourish or drain our prana. The thoughts we think, actions we take, situations we put ourselves in and people we align ourselves with can also fuel or deplete us. Choose wisely.

When you eat junk you feel like crap. When you add in nutrient-dense foods, you feel powerful and energized. You may not associate it immediately but little-by-little as you make changes, you will become more in-tune with your body. To stay strong and healthy, speed recovery time and feel fantastic, superfoods are your ticket. To increase inflammation, slow healing time, decrease strength and lower performance ability, eat lots of junk foods.

Everyone is a superhero on some level. Whether you are training for sports or battling a disease, it is all relative and we all deserve to be our best. Greatness starts with how we eat. You can train for hours a day and even stretch daily, but if you eat the Standard American Diet (SAD) of processed foods, you are decreasing your warrior strength and limiting your highest potential.

You'll notice we're not even going to talk about weight loss. Although weight loss is certainly a side effect of an anti-inflammatory superfood diet, this is not my focus. My goal was, and still is, to create healing. I have lost some weight along the way, but allowing my body to heal and settle in to its natural set point was the key. The focus feels positive (gain health) instead of negative (lose weight). The term "diet" has gotten a bad rap. The Flexible Warrior program is not one you'll go on or off of. I don't want you to be on a roller coaster ride. Make small, sustainable changes that fuel your life force and you'll never have to feel guilty or count calories again. It's as easy as taking out the garbage.

What's Your Kryptonite? What's Your Superfood?

One person's magic potion is another person's kryptonite. There is not one single list of foods that will work for everyone. For me, coffee, alcohol and dark chocolate are all kryptonite if I have them daily. These foods can trigger migraines, pain, inflammation and suffering for me. For others, these foods and drinks could be magical elixirs that energize and nourish.

You intuitively already know what your kryptonite foods are. But sometimes we are addicted to the very foods that hurt us the most. Like an alcoholic, you might even be in denial. It took me six years to give up coffee, but it was worth it. When I drank coffee daily, it was a serious source of inflammation. Now I have it every once in a while as a treat and it is exhilarating. Coffee turned from being my kryptonite to now being the superfood it was meant to be, enjoyed in moderation. Drinking high quality organic coffee is a critical part of the equation.

To me, a superfood is any food that energizes, heals and nourishes your prana. Fresh juices, green smoothies, raw fruits and veggies make me feel light and energized. For you, green juice may make you gag or make your blood sugar unstable. Maybe your superfoods are proteins like meat, yogurt and eggs. Since we all have unique chemistry, how our body responds to different foods also varies. As the saying goes, "One man's potion is another man's poison."

Food as Medicine

It's now believed that chronic inflammation is the root cause for many debilitating diseases. Instead of changing our diet, we pop pills, which often causes adverse side effects and certainly doesn't fix the root cause: inflammation. Using food as medicine reduces inflammation, decreases illness and increases vitality.

Beyond stretching, massage and self-care, the best thing you can do to improve your flexibility and recovery is to take out the garbage foods and add in nutrient-dense, high quality anti-inflammatory super foods. You may feel more energized and flexible within a few days or it may take a year until the inflammation starts to fade and the flexibility and power kicks in. Consistency is the key. Don't give up!

One of the most selfish things we can do is eat junk food and not take care of ourselves, which ultimately exposes us to a greater chance of illness and disease. When we're sickly, it affects our family and every person who comes in to contact with us. When we're healthy we can accomplish great things. We have energy to share. In that sense, self-care is one of the most selfless things you can do.

Healthy foods can be more expensive, but there are many resources available to help you buy organic on a budget. Plus, the money you'll save on doctor bills and time off work for sick days will save you money in the long run.

What Does Food Have To Do With Flexibility?

Everyone knows that a diet full of processed foods is causing the obesity crisis, but few people realize that our dietary choices also have an effect on health as a whole, including pain and flexibility. The Standard American Diet is inflammatory which can lead to stiffness, reduced range of motion and decreased flexibility.

Foods that trigger inflammation include refined grains, processed breads, chips, crackers, deli meats, sweets like cake, cookies, muffins, polyunsaturated cooking oils (corn, sunflower, safflower), alcoholic beverages, trans fats in fast foods and baked goods, fake butter like margarine and food additives and preservatives like MSG, food coloring and artificial flavors.

Filling up on foods like fruits, vegetables, whole grains and moderate amounts of healthy fats and clean proteins are less inflammatory. Research shows that foods high in antioxidants and phytonutrients help neutralize free radical damage which also reduces inflammation. Foods like nuts, seeds, olive oil, legumes and many spices like turmeric, ginger and cinnamon are great choices. Natural sweeteners like honey, maple syrup and dried fruits are fine in moderation.

A healthy diet full of antioxidants and phytonutrients will reduce inflammation, decrease pain and improve your overall health and vitality. It's the simple things like adequate sleep, hydration, deep breathing, reducing stress, getting moderate exercise and eating healthy that are the most effective at reducing inflammation.

There are many resources on reducing inflammation. Some of my favorites are functional medicine doctors: Mark Hyman, Susan Blum, Amy Myers, Josh Axe and Lissa Rankin. Research your specific health concerns and find additional information about healing with diet. Here are six tips to begin reducing chronic inflammation:

1) Eat less animal protein. Choose grass-fed, organic meats when possible. Join the meatless Monday revolution! Find a local organic farmer.
2) Eat more organic veggies, especially leafy greens like kale and spinach. Start each meal with a salad for phytonutrients, vitamins and minerals.
3) Eat less processed foods. Eat more fresh, whole foods.
4) Take a chill pill. Rest, stretch and relax more. When our bodies are in a state of constant stress we are unable to repair. Get 8 hours of sleep per night.
5) Drink plain water. Sugary beverages increase inflammation. Plain water is superior for hydration. If you need electrolytes, try coconut water. Most sports drinks are filled with sugar, artificial colors and flavors. Diet soda is toxic and dehydrating!
6) Practice more self-care. Breathe, meditate, stretch and center your mind. Avoid toxic relationships as much as toxic foods. Make time for stillness. Be open to new experiences and ways of eating and thinking.

<u>Flexible Warrior Diet Rules:</u>

The #1 diet rule is this: if it makes you feel good, eat it! But the food can't just feel good while you're eating it, only to later cause you to crash and burn. It must make you feel good during *and* after eating it to fit this rule. Remember, it's not about restriction and eating a perfect diet. It's an experiment, so there is no guilt. Use your intuition and common sense. The less you stress about eating and enjoy your food, the less disease and inflammation you will create and the more flexible and resilient you will become! Flexibility is power!

Three Simple Rules:

1) If it makes you feel good, eat it.

2) If it makes you feel bad, skip it.

3) Keep it simple, stress free and enjoyable.

1) If it makes you feel good, eat it.

Superfoods are hot right now. Chia seeds, raw cacao, kale and goji berries. I love superfoods blended into smoothies! But these trendy superfoods are not the only foods that are super for your health. Your superfoods might be grass-fed meat, organic eggs, or even whole grain bread. Each of us has unique chemistry, genetics and history. Our superfoods and kryptonite foods are different. The biggest goal is to get back to basics, eating and enjoying a variety of fresh, local, real foods and increasing awareness of how you feel after you eat.

2) If it makes you feel bad, skip it!

This rule sounds like common sense, but why do so many people eat junk food that makes them sick and feel bad? I think part of the problem is that we don't associate our aches, pains, illnesses and digestive issues with our diet.

If you experience stomach issues or have other health problems, it might be time to consider an elimination diet to see if food could be triggering or exacerbating your health issues. Sometimes taking a break from a certain food (like dairy or gluten) can be eye-opening! Suddenly the symptoms disappear that you didn't even associate with food.

You may be in denial that coffee, sugar, gluten or alcohol are causing you to feel less than your best. But deep inside you know the truth! This is your life! You have one shot! Isn't it worth going without a few addictive foods for a while to see how good you can feel? With an elimination diet, you remove suspicious foods for a short period of time and then add them back in to see how you feel.

If you think a detox seems too hard, consider that the truly hard things in life are way more uncomfortable than giving up coffee or sugar for two weeks, the rewards have the ability to save you so much pain, time and money in the long run and nothing worthwhile is ever easy. Enduring a little discomfort is how we grow stronger and more flexible and resilient. Doing hard things is the path to transformation.

3) Keep it simple, balanced and stress free.

For about 20 years (the 80s to 90s) I drank Diet Coke and ate fat-free everything. Yet somehow I couldn't lose weight, was always exhausted, had acne and got migraines. I didn't put two and two together. It took me years to understand that what I was (and wasn't) eating was causing so many problems. Because of that experience, I'm skeptical of new diet trends and products. I don't jump into the latest craze but I do try to JERF (Just Eat Real Food). No matter if you are gluten-free, paleo or vegan, keep it fresh, local and simple and you'll be on the right path.

JERF

I learned the term JERF from Sean Croxton at Underground Wellness. We are all super busy and the last thing we need is to stress about time-consuming recipes and expensive shopping lists. When you JERF, it's simple and stress-free. You limit stress-inducing inflammatory foods and you increase clean, whole, real foods.

Real food is not chemicalized, processed, stripped of nutrients and enhanced with flavors and additives. Real food is not genetically modified, packaged in colorful boxes and shipped halfway around the world. Real food won't run a commercial during the Super Bowl featuring a rock star. Real food is perfect just as it is. It doesn't need to be modified, processed or packaged. Get back to basics and JERF.

Read food labels!

The FDA regulates food labels and they are constantly changing the guidelines so it can be very confusing and often misleading. Of course, if you're staying gluten-free and non-GMO, you'll want to read your food labels carefully. Beyond serving size, calories and health claims, what you really want to pay attention to is the ingredient list.

The general rule of thumb is, if you can't read it, don't eat it! Avoid health claims like "natural" or "low sugar" because they are usually marketing technique red flags to persuade you to eat something processed. Steer clear of unfamiliar additives and preservatives. Stick to ingredient lists that you can read and understand. For example, natural peanut butter contains: peanuts and sea salt. Easy. Regular peanut butter contains: peanuts, sugar, hydrogenated oils, monoglycerides and diglycerides. Many additives and preservatives are inflammatory and toxic.

Train yourself to look beyond health claims and choose foods with short and simple ingredient lists. This one simple tool can make a big difference in the quality of your foods.

Isn't an Egg an Egg?

What's the difference between wild-caught salmon and farm-raised? They look the same, so they must have the same nutrients, right? Studies have compared factory farm-raised fish and meat to wild-caught fish and grass-fed meats and the nutritional values are extremely different. Factory farm-raised animals don't get the natural diet they would eat in the wild, which affects the nutrients and quality of the meat.

Organic apples versus GMO (Genetically Modified Organism) apples have different nutrient values, as does kale from your grocery store versus organic from your local farmer. Fruits and veggies can lose nutrients from over-farmed soil, aging and exposure as they are shipped across the country. Local organic farm-grown veggies have prana.

Three years ago, I began getting veggies and eggs from a local farmer (Oak Spring Farm in Freeland, Maryland) through a CSA (Community Supported Agriculture) farm. The variety is so fun, the quality is amazing and supporting a local farmer I trust with my food is very rewarding. Before the CSA, I would buy the same veggies week after week. The quality was hit or miss and since it was shipped across the country, it was rarely fresh. These days I'm always experimenting and trying something new. In addition, knowing these superfood veggies are fresh, nutrient-dense and toxin-free, I'm getting more bang for my buck.

We could devote a whole chapter to eggs and the difference between organic, free-range, pastured and regular eggs. I challenge you to pick up some pastured eggs from your farmers market and do your own comparison to regular grocery store eggs. They look similar on the outside, but differ greatly in color and taste. Nutritional studies comparing eggs prove the nutrients vary greatly depending on how the chickens were raised and what they were fed. Find a local farmer and buy organic pastured eggs if possible. They have a higher content of healthy Omega-3 fats and other nutrients. If you get the chance to pick up your eggs from a CSA farm, don't forget to thank the chickens!

You spend so much time and money on trainers, gadgets and gear, it is worth spending a few extra dollars on the fuel that nourishes every cell of your body! A simple place to start is the Dirty Dozen and The Clean Fifteen lists from the Environmental Working Group (EWG). Carry the lists with you to the grocery store. If you can't afford to buy all organic, just avoid the *Dirty Dozen* and buy organic from that list. You can feel safer buying non-organic from the *Clean Fifteen* list.

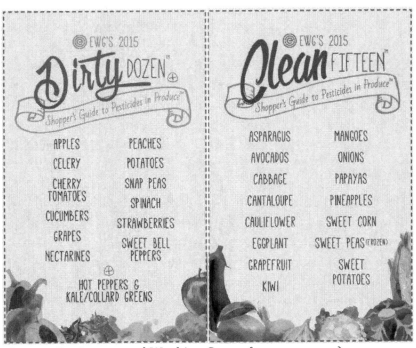

Source: Environmental Working Group (www.ewg.org)

Celery is one of the most toxic, pesticide-treated veggies. When I was shopping for Christmas dinner, my store was out of organic celery. Yes, it would have been easier, faster and more convenient to just buy the regular celery. No one in my family would have known the difference, but there was no way I was feeding my family chemicals for Christmas! So I made an extra stop on one of the busiest shopping days of the year. If it had been onions or avocados I would have bought the non-organic, but non-organic celery is like spraying pesticides on your stuffing.

Foods That Increase Inflammation:

- Sugar
- Artificial sweeteners
- MSG, artificial flavors and preservatives
- GMO fruits and vegetables
- High fructose corn syrup
- Processed, refined grains
- Corn and soy
- Margarine and fake butter spreads
- Gluten
- Grains
- Bad fats (hydrogenated or partially hydrogenated oil)
- Alcohol
- Factory farm meats and farm-raised fish
- Processed meats (like deli meats and hot dogs)
- Fast food
- Non-organic dairy

You may not be sensitive to all of the items on this list, so don't feel like you have to eliminate them all from your diet. You may also be sensitive to foods that aren't on this list, but these are the usual offenders. An elimination diet may be a worthwhile experiment. Temporarily removing suspicious foods from your diet, then adding them back in, allows you to target foods that are causing you distress.

Be aware of your Omega-6/Omega-3 balance. The Standard American Diet is high in inflammatory Omega-6 fatty acids (grains, processed foods and vegetable oils) and low in anti-inflammatory Omega-3s (from foods like fatty fish, extra virgin olive oil and walnuts). The balance between these essential fatty acids is so important. With concerns about mercury in fish and quality supplements, refer to expert sources like Dr. Mark Hyman and Dr. Josh Axe.

<u>Anti-Inflammatory choices:</u>

- Low-fat organic dairy like kefir and unsweetened organic yogurt (if you are not dairy sensitive); stick to real organic grass-fed butter
- Organic grass-fed/grass-finished, pasture-raised meats
- Wild-caught fatty fish (like salmon)
- Fresh herbs (like parsley and rosemary) & spices (like ginger, cinnamon and turmeric)
- Organic, whole grains (if you're not grain sensitive)
- Organic fruit (especially berries and cherries)
- Organic vegetables (especially leafy greens like kale)
- Raw, local honey
- Seaweed and algae (like kelp and spirulina)
- Green tea (unsweetened)
- Extra virgin olive oil and organic coconut oil
- Omega-3 or pastured eggs
- Bone broth soups and stews (organic, grass-fed bones)

Food or Pills?

What you eat can have a powerful effect on reducing inflammation and pain. An interesting study found that Omega-3 fatty acid supplements were an effective alternative treatment to anti-inflammatory NSAID drugs. There is an abundance of information from functional medicine doctors about foods that fight inflammation including chia seeds, kimchi, coconut oil, kale and turmeric.

Superfood expert David Wolfe healed himself of chronic pain with yoga and food after he was told by doctors he had a mechanical problem in his spine. His approach to anti-inflammatory foods incorporates raw foods, superfoods, superherbs and supplements like MSM, Vitamin C, medicinal mushrooms and mangosteen. One of David's favorite natural anti-inflammatories is fresh vegetable juice including cucumber, celery and fennel, which has hydrating and healing properties.

Although bone broth might not be the first thing that comes to mind when you think of superfoods, it has so many healing and anti-inflammatory qualities. For me, juices and smoothies are great in the warmer months, but when it's cold, bone broth, soups and stews are best, especially when filled with anti-inflammatory veggies and herbs like celery, parsley, kale, carrots, onions and garlic.

Some of my favorite references for anti-inflammatory foods are Julie Daniluk's *Meals That Heal Inflammation* and *The Autoimmune Paleo Cookbook* by Mickey Trescott. Julie's book is packed with scientific references and delicious recipes that are free from inflammatory triggers and full of healing properties. Mickey's cookbook is gorgeous and filled with beautiful and healthy paleo recipes.

Incorporating healing foods can help to reduce inflammation and pain flare-ups and speed the healing process from injuries, illness and even surgery. As the pain and stiffness from chronic inflammation decreases, your range of motion, freedom of movement and flexibility will increase.

Superfoods

Adding in superfoods is super easy! If you replace your fast food breakfast with a superfood smoothie, that is a huge step in the right direction! Look for smoothie recipes on Pinterest and follow *Simple Green Smoothies* on Instagram.

There are more and more superfoods on the market so experiment and see what appeals to you. The only rule is that you eat what makes *you* feel good. Apples from the orchard a few miles from your house may be a better superfood for you than expensive berries shipped halfway around the planet.

Here are 12 of my favorite superfoods to get you started:

Chia Seeds are a powerful little seed, high in antioxidants and Omega-3 fatty acids. A friend of mine fueled his entire marathon on chia seeds alone! The first time I was introduced to chia I was at a Yoga for Veterans training for *Semper Fidelis Health & Wellness*. The class leader, a former marine, made a jar of gelled-up chia seeds and gave us all shots, like we were in a bar. He explained they were a superfood for warriors, so I have been hooked ever since. The biggest downfall with chia is that it tends to get stuck in my teeth so I also buy them ground. Chia seeds help the body maintain hydration and are a great energy source.

Goji Berries are known as the longevity food and are packed with powerful phytonutrients and antioxidants that boost performance and energy. They are my favorite pre-race snack and they are much healthier than gummy bears! They are also a complete protein.

Sprouted Grains like Ezekiel brand bread, superfood cereal and Kashi brand sprouted grain cereal are great options for nutrient-dense fast food. If gluten is an issue, beware that many of these products are not gluten-free so read labels carefully. The breads are often found in the frozen section of a grocery store. I keep my bread in the freezer and pull out a few slices so it can last for weeks.

Green Tea is high in antioxidants and polyphenols. It does contain caffeine which can energize and awaken you, but the amount of caffeine is small compared to coffee, so it rarely causes a jittery buzz. Green tea is shown to reduce the growth of cancer cells and lower your risk for infection and Type 2 diabetes.

Coconut Water, Coconut Milk and Coconut Oil are all regulars in my recipes. Coconut water is the best electrolyte sports drink with no added colors, sugars or flavors. Coconut milk is a great source of healthy fat and helps reduce inflammation. Coconut oil is the best replacement for processed oils and has many other healthy uses beyond cooking. Check out *101 Uses of Coconut Oil* by Wellness Mama and *77 Coconut Oil Uses & Cures* by Dr. Josh Axe.

Leafy greens are high in chlorophyll (pure life force) which helps oxygenate the blood, increase circulation and speed healing. Green juices and smoothies help you boost the amount of greens you to consume. Raw greens are super high in vitamins, minerals and enzymes. Kale is getting all the attention these days but spinach, collards, bok choy and beet greens are all amazing.

Blueberries are high in antioxidants and have anti-inflammatory qualities. Buy frozen organic blueberries for convenience. My favorite purple power smoothie is blueberries, almond or coconut milk, Sunwarrior protein, Navitas Naturals Superfruit powder and a little raw honey. A berry smoothie is healthy fast food. It takes just a few minutes to prepare and you can put it in a mason jar to go!

Raw Honey is unprocessed and unfiltered and it's the best sweetener, in my opinion, because it's delicious and has nutritional value. Since it's unfiltered, it has a thick consistency and a bit of a funky smell. Raw honey is very high in antioxidants, enzymes, vitamins and minerals. Use raw honey in your tea or smoothies.

Hemp Seeds are the most nutritious seeds in the world and are high in Omega fatty acids, protein, vitamins and minerals. Lately, my salads and smoothies are not complete without a sprinkle of hemp seeds or a scoop of hemp protein.

Algae (spirulina and chlorella) are complete proteins that are easy to absorb and are packed with vitamins, minerals, essential fatty acids and everything you need to build plant-based strength and endurance. When I'm making a green smoothie, I love adding a scoop of spirulina for an added boost of nutrients. But don't add it to your berry or chocolate smoothies or they will turn a brown color that isn't as visually appealing as vibrant green.

Seaweed is very high in mineral content and chlorophyll which helps oxygenate the blood and boost tissue repair. I love seaweed salad but you can also pick up dulse, nori wraps or kelp and add them to a tossed salad or eat them as a snack.

Sprouts can supercharge your salads with protein, which helps with tissue repair, healing and recovery. When a seed sprouts, it transforms to become a plant and this new state allows its nutrients to be better digested and absorbed. Sprouts are nutrient-dense little powerhouses of energy. Pick up various bean sprouts in the refrigerated area of your produce aisle.

Walnuts are high in Omega-3 fats and are a great anti-inflammatory snack. Soaking nuts in salt water removes the enzyme inhibitor (phytic acid) that's in the skin of the nut. Phytic acid blocks absorption of nutrients and makes nuts harder to digest. Buy raw organic nuts when possible and soak them overnight, rinse and dry them before eating.

Avocado is high in fat, which scares people, but the healthy fats and nutrients in an avocado are very powerful and filling. Yes, guacamole is awesome, but I also love smashing an avocado onto my Ezekiel toast with some sea salt, having it with morning eggs, making a green goddess salad dressing or adding it to a green smoothie for a creamy texture. If you have a high-powered blender, you can use the avocado seed, which is also packed with fiber and nutrients.

Cacao might be my favorite superfood. Who doesn't love chocolate?! Raw cacao is high in minerals like magnesium, which is a natural muscle relaxant and is delicious in smoothies, desserts and protein bars. An easy energizing, anti-inflammatory smoothie is raw cacao, a frozen banana, cinnamon, coconut milk and a little raw honey. Try this concoction instead of a latte and see how energized you feel!

Spices like ginger, cinnamon and turmeric can lower inflammation and reduce pain. You can take them in supplement form or add them to your favorite recipes. I sprinkle ginger and cinnamon on everything from toast and oatmeal to smoothies and tea. I am still learning to experiment with turmeric. A friend of mine recently turned me on to the calming tea she saw on The Dr. Oz show with turmeric, cinnamon, ginger, honey and almond milk.

Consider that some of the most amazing superherbs grow in our own backyard. Dandelion is so hardy, it can grow through a crack in our sidewalk. But instead of eating it, we kill it with toxic chemicals. Dandelion is shown to be a natural anti-inflammatory and offers support for our liver, kidney and gallbladder. If you spray your lawn with pesticides and fertilizers, don't eat the dandelions in your yard. Once again, some of the best things in life are free.

Including superfoods and superherbs in our diet every day can supercharge energy and boost health. Superfoods are the most nutrient-dense foods on the planet and although our ancestors ate them for thousands of years, they are often forgotten in modern times because they were not mass produced and heavily marketed. Recently, superfoods have become much more available and most grocery stores now carry a wide selection. Choosing superfoods over junk foods can completely transform your diet. Experiment and find the superfoods you enjoy that make you feel fantastic.

The topic of protein is highly debated. There is a recent trend toward higher animal protein, paleo and ancestral diets. There is also a trend toward vegan and vegetable-based diets, even among high-level athletes. The amino acids found in protein are essential in each cell and are the building block for a strong, lean body. Protein is a personal choice. Pay attention to how you feel after eating different sources of protein. Are you energized or sleepy? Do you feel strong or fatigued?

Remember the type and quality of the protein you choose can make a huge difference. When possible, choose high-quality organic, free-range, grass-fed meats. Not only is pasture, grass-fed farming better for our environment, the meats are also healthier. They are higher in Omega-3 fatty acids, which reduce inflammation.

As a flexitarian, I personally eat meat more as a side dish and load up on veggies and plant-based proteins. Vegetables are actually a great protein source. I was shocked when I first heard that pound per pound, spinach has more protein than meat. Bear in mind that a pound of spinach is quite a lot of greens to consume. Most people need less meat than they are consuming. An average serving size is the palm of your hand.

Vegan Protein Sources

- Nuts and seeds like walnuts, almonds and chia
- Protein powders like hemp, pea and rice protein
- Leafy greens like spinach and kale
- Grains like quinoa and rice
- Beans like lentils, black beans and chick peas
- Soy like tofu and edamame
- Superfoods like spirulina and goji berries

All these vegetable sources of protein should be non-GMO and organic when possible. Boost the protein to your smoothies by adding hemp seeds, nut butter, chia or flax seeds, spirulina or a high quality vegan protein powder.

The topic of gluten is another highly debated, controversial subject. If you have Celiac disease or gluten intolerance, you should remove gluten from your diet. Many experts feel that a wheat-free, gluten-free diet is beneficial for everyone. However, because of the gluten-free trend, there are many products on the market now that are free from gluten, but are full of other potential hazards like GMO corn, soy and sugar. Just because a product is gluten-free does not necessarily mean it's healthy. Beware of processed, gluten-free junk foods.

I recently read an entertaining perspective on the gluten-free trend. The eye-catching graphic said, "Cocaine is gluten-free." The point of the article is to be aware of diet and marketing trends and of big food companies jumping in to profit. In other words, gluten-free or not, limit processed foods in general and JERF.

Anti-Inflammatory and Adaptogenic Herbs & Supplements

As we discussed earlier, there are many different herbs and supplements that have excellent anti-inflammatory properties. You should always check with your doctor first, but some herbs and supplements to consider are turmeric, ginger, boswellia, MSM, Vitamin C, medicinal mushrooms, Omega-3 fish oil and mangosteen.

I prefer to get most of my vitamins, minerals and nutrients from high quality food instead of supplements, but it's challenging due to depleted soil. Your needs are different, but taking a high quality multi-vitamin and mineral supplement along with probiotics for gut health, digestive enzymes, magnesium and extra Vitamin D and C have made a big difference in my energy and overall health.

Supplementing with magnesium in particular really helped me with both muscular pain and headaches.

Magnesium is responsible for over 300 biochemical reactions in the body. Studies show around 80 percent of Americans are magnesium deficient, due to depleted soil and poor diet.

The top 10 magnesium-rich foods listed by Dr. Axe are spinach, swiss chard, pumpkin seeds, yogurt, kefir, almonds, black beans, avocado, figs, dark chocolate and bananas. Making a smoothie with raw cacao, yogurt and a banana is a great magnesium-rich breakfast or post-workout recovery snack.

Be aware of toxins in many supplements. Taking cheap supplements is not only a waste of money, it can also be counterproductive and detrimental to your health. Invest in quality supplements from reputable sources.

Adaptogenic Herbs

Adaptogenic herbs work by helping to balance your adrenal system, which is in charge of how you respond to and manage stress, helping you better cope with anxiety and fatigue. They are called "adaptogens" because they have the ability to adapt their function based on each person's individual needs.

During my treatment for Lyme, I mistakenly used coffee and sugar to help me get through the day. If I knew then what I know now I wouldn't have put additional stress on my system with these stimulants. Had I used adaptogenic herbs instead, I may have saved myself years of pain and fatigue.

I know I'm not the only one. Millions of people reach for coffee and cupcakes every single day. If you have an illness or infection, your immune system is already stressed trying to fight and heal. Don't make it worse by eating a diet full of inflammatory stimulants, sugar and chemicals. Also, chronic stress can be as detrimental to your health as an infection so make lifestyle changes to reduce stress if you need to.

Adaptogenic herbs can have an amazing and powerful effect, but working with a doctor or health care provider is advised since everyone is different. Some adaptogenic herbs to look into include: ginseng, eleuthero, ashwagandha, rhodiola rosea, astragalus and schizandra berry.

Better Carb-Loading and Race Recovery

The day before a race, instead of choosing processed pasta or a bagel with jam, experiment with a sprouted grain or organic sourdough bread with almond butter, cinnamon and raw honey. Organic, whole grain oatmeal with almond or coconut milk is a great option. You can try gluten-free rice noodles loaded with vegetables and a little olive oil, lemon and sea salt. A simple sweet potato is loaded with high quality carbs and nutrients plus it has natural anti-inflammatory properties.

Start carb-loading with your favorite superfoods the week before your race. Load-up on green or fruit smoothies, and add in superfoods like chia seeds, raw honey, spinach, cacao, goji berries and coconut water. Eat lots of hydrating, nutrient-dense organic fruits and vegetables. Try some high quality, fresh vegetable and fruit juices.

Opt for a healthy magnesium-rich, post-race recovery smoothie with a banana, berries, cacao, coconut water, almond or other nut milk, organic yogurt and a high quality vegan protein powder. Experiment well in advance of your race day to see what foods boost your performance, supercharge your energy and speed your recovery.

Drinking

I hate to be a buzzkill, but drinking alcoholic beverages can significantly increase inflammation. Just to confuse the issue, there are studies that show moderate drinking can be healthy and reduce the risk of cardiovascular disease.

The saying that "One man's poison is another man's cure" holds true. It's ironic because alcoholic drinks can feel like somewhat of a superfood for some people, temporarily making them feel energized and happy. For others, alcohol almost immediately makes us feel awful. I fall into the latter category. Alcohol is kryptonite to me, so I rarely drink. It took me about 30 years to really embrace not drinking (that story is a whole other book).

Drinking is a personal choice, but we all know it can have dangerous side effects and addictive qualities. Your best bet for alcohol consumption is moderation. Red wine is high in the anti-inflammatory compound called resveratrol, so try an organic red wine instead of hard liquor or a sugary cocktail. Many bars are now serving fresh fruit and vegetable juice cocktails and non-alcoholic mocktails. Cheers!

The Flexible Warrior Diet

To summarize, the Flexible Warrior diet offers a lot of freedom and variety. The simple goal is to eat less inflammatory junk foods and increase anti-inflammatory superfoods. What and how you eat can affect your recovery, flexibility, performance and of course your overall health. The goal is not about restriction and perfection.. Drink more water and less sugary beverages. When possible, choose more organic, locally-grown vegetables, pastured eggs, grass-fed meats and wild-caught fish. It's realistic and practical.

Conclusion

The Flexible Warrior approach is something I learned and created over 25 years. The balance between strength and willpower and flexibility and chillpower came with lots of practice and patience. If you're a warrior-type with lots of willpower, adding in chillpower, recovery and flexibility can bring peace and more balance.

Finding balance in this hectic world may not feel natural or easy. Taking time to breathe and stretch might feel like a complete waste of time. My hope is that, after reading this book, you will be more willing to invest more in self-care, stretching and healing foods.

Flexibility is a great strength... in how we think, how we eat, how we exercise and how we react when things don't go as planned or when we're blind-sided by life. Embrace the obstacles as learning experiences. Our wounds are often our greatest teachers.

Most warrior-types are willing to do many uncomfortable things and spend a lot of money on whatever improves their success, performance and productivity. Although stretching, self-care and healthy eating can support all these goals, they seem to be last on the list for most people. The best self-care methods are often free... fresh air, clean water and quality rest. It's time to get back to basics.

More and more, my grocery bill and self-care appointments are my biggest expenses. I'd rather spend my money on good food, a massage and quality supplements than on doctor's bills and prescription drugs.

We each need to find our own sense of balance between strength and flexibility, power and peace, stop and go and cookies and kale.

"Don't worry about the future; know that worrying is as effective as trying to solve an algebra equation by chewing bubblegum. The real troubles in your life are apt to be things that never crossed your worried mind; the kind that blindside you at 4PM on some idle Tuesday."

- Baz Luhrmann, "Everybody's Free (To Wear Sunscreen)"

Appendix

10 Questions To Be A More Flexible Warrior

Grab your journal or a piece of paper and jot down the answers to these questions. Post sticky notes on your refrigerator or at your desk. Set reminders on your phone or add a new category to your training schedule. Awareness and taking little steps can make a big difference over time.

1) Where in your life can you be more flexible?
2) What can you let go of that is not aligned with your values or no longer serves your higher purpose?
3) Where in your life can you be more of a warrior? How can you practice more discipline or take more action?
4) What areas of your life could benefit from more willpower? What steps are you willing to take to get what you want? What obstacles are in your way? How can you overcome those obstacles?
5) What areas of your life could benefit from more chillpower? Are there times you feel like you are swimming upstream? If so, how can you relax more and go with the flow?
6) What can you do today, this week and this year to incorporate more self-care? How can you take better care of your mind, body and spirit?
7) What kinds of stretching and flexibility training can you add to your schedule? When? Where? How do you think it will benefit you?
8) What foods are kryptonite to you? How do they negatively affect you? What foods can replace them?
9) What foods fuel your prana? How do they make you feel? How can you increase these foods?
10) How can you achieve more balance in your life? What can you do to feel stronger and more resilient?

References

Chapter 1: Willpower

-"Do Hard Things | The Rebelution." 2013.
<http://therebelution.com/books/do-hard-things/>
-"Knights of Heroes Foundation."
http://www.knightsofheroes.org/
-"Spartan Race: Obstacle Races." 2015. www.spartan.com
-"Tough Mudder: Mud Run | Obstacle Races." 2014
www.toughmudder.com

Chapter 2: Chillpower

-"One Word." 2011. <http://getoneword.com/>
-"We Are Marshall." 2007.
<http://wearemarshalldvd.warnerbros.com/>

Chapter 3: Self-care for Warriors

-"Does Exercise Weaken Immune System? - Livestrong.com."
2010. <http://www.livestrong.com/article/331034-does-exercise-
weaken-immune-system/>
-"What Happens to Muscles During Exercise? - FitStar ." 2014.
<http://fitstar.com/happens-muscles-exercise-2/>
-"Reducing Whole Body Inflammation? - Ask Dr. Weil." 2011.
<http://www.drweil.com/drw/u/QAA401013/Reducing-Whole-
Body-Inflammation.html>
-"The Healing Foods Diet - DrAxe.com." 2014.
<http://draxe.com/healing-diet/>
-"The Best Diet for Recovering From a Sports Injury ..." 2011.
<http://www.livestrong.com/article/412947-the-best-diet-for-
recovering-from-a-sports-injury/>
-"7 Foods That Fight Inflammation - Guide to Managing ..."
2014. <http://www.everydayhealth.com/health-
report/rheumatoid-arthritis-pictures/foods-that-fight-
inflammation.aspx>

-"Treatment of Fibromyalgia - Dr. Weil." 2008.
<http://www.drweil.com/drw/u/ART02975/Treatment-of-Fibromyalgia.html>

-"Reiki - What You Need to Know - Alternative Medicine."
2007. <http://altmedicine.about.com/od/reiki/a/reiki.htm>

-"Magnesium: The Missing Link to Better Health - Mercola."
2013.
<http://articles.mercola.com/sites/articles/archive/2013/12/08/magnesium-health-benefits.aspx>

-"Natural Calm—Anti Stress - Natural Vitality." 2014. 13
<https://naturalvitality.com/natural-calm/>

-"Ancient Minerals | Ultra Pure Magnesium Oil," 2008.
<http://www.ancient-minerals.com/>

-"The Magnesium Miracle | Dr Carolyn Dean MD ND." 2009.
<http://drcarolyndean.com/magnesium_miracle/>

-"Arnica in Homeopathy - WebMD." 2011.
<http://www.webmd.com/vitamins-and-supplements/arnica>

-"Traumeel." 2005. 23 Jan. 2015 <http://www.traumeel.com/>

-"Health Journeys: Guided Meditation | Guided Imagery "
<http://www.healthjourneys.com/>

-"Dry needling - Wikipedia, the free encyclopedia." 2006.
<http://en.wikipedia.org/wiki/Dry_needling>

-"The remarkable health benefits of Epsom salt baths ..." 2013.
<http://www.naturalnews.com/042753_epsom_salt_baths_remarkable_health_benefits_detoxificatin_technique.html>

-"Magnesium: The Missing Link to Better Health - Mercola."
2013.
<http://articles.mercola.com/sites/articles/archive/2013/12/08/magnesium-health-benefits.aspx>

-"Ice bath - Wikipedia, the free encyclopedia." 2006.
<http://en.wikipedia.org/wiki/Ice_bath>

-"People, We've Got to Stop Icing Injuries. We Were Wrong ..."
2013. <http://www.mobilitywod.com/2012/08/people-weve-got-to-stop-icing-we-were-wrong-sooo-wrong/>

-"Thai Yoga Massage - Yoga Journal." 2014.
<http://www.yogajournal.com/article/practice-section/get-in-touch/>

-"Benefits of Thai Yoga Massage | LIVESTRONG.COM." 2010. <http://www.livestrong.com/article/135880-benefits-thai-yoga-massage/>

-"Reflexology - Dr. Weil's Wellness Therapies - DrWeil.com." 2010. <http://www.drweil.com/drw/u/ART00546/Reflexology-Dr-Weil-Wellness-Therapies.html>

-"YTU Therapy Balls w/Tote | Yoga Tune Up®." 2013. <https://www.yogatuneup.com/ytu-therapy-balls-wtote>

-"Myofascial trigger point - Wikipedia, the free encyclopedia." 2014. <http://en.wikipedia.org/wiki/Myofascial_trigger_point>

-"TheStick.net - Neck Pain, Leg pain, Back Pain, Arm Pain." <http://www.thestick.net/>

-"Article - Using Foam Rollers by Michael Boyle - Perform Better." 2014. <http://www.performbetter.com/webapp/wcs/stores/servlet/PBOnePieceView?storeId=10151&catalogId=10751&pagename=225>

-"Trigger Point Performance Therapy." 2012. <https://www.tptherapy.com/>

-"OPTP Posture Ball | Shop OPTP.com." 2013. <http://www.optp.com/Posture-Ball>

-"Self Massage Therapy Balls - Yoga Tune Up." 2013. <https://www.yogatuneup.com/self-massage-therapy-balls-programs>

-"MobilityWOD | All human beings should be able to perform ..." 2010. <http://www.mobilitywod.com/>

-"Dara Torres Bio - Ki-Hara Resistance Stretching - Innovative ..." 2012. <http://ki-hara.com/Athletes-darabio.php>

-"About Intrinsic Health Systems." 2008. <http://www.intrinsichealthsystems.com/about-us/>

-"Mashing - Ki-Hara Resistance Stretching - Innovative Body ..." 2012. <http://ki-hara.com/mashing.php>

-"Lack of Sleep and the Immune System - WebMD." 2010. 26 <http://www.webmd.com/sleep-disorders/excessive-sleepiness-10/immune-system-lack-of-sleep>

-"Sleep & Athletic Performance - National Sleep Foundation." 2014. <http://sleepfoundation.org/sleep-news/sleep-athletic-performance-and-recovery>

-"Sleeping Tips & Tricks - National Sleep Foundation." 2014.
<http://sleepfoundation.org/sleep-tools-tips/healthy-sleep-tips>

-"WaterCure | The Miracles of Water to Cure Diseases."
<http://www.watercure.com/>

-"Foods for Leg Cramps | LIVESTRONG.COM." 2010.
<http://www.livestrong.com/article/116308-foods-prevent-leg-
cramps/>

-"How does the BioMat compare to far infrared ray saunas ..."
2011. <http://www.biomat.com/how-does-the-biomat-compare-
to-far-infrared-ray-saunas-and-domes/>

-"Health Benefits of a Sauna | Dr. Julian Whitaker." 2014.
<http://www.drwhitaker.com/health-benefits-of-a-sauna>

-"Bio-individuality - Institute for Integrative Nutrition." 2014.
<http://www.integrativenutrition.com/blog/2013/03/notes-
from-iin%E2%80%99s-founder-why-it%E2%80%99s-ok-to-quit-
being-vegan-or-macrobiotic>

-"Perfect Breathing | Welcome to your perfect breath!" 2006.
26 <http://www.perfectbreathing.com/>

-"The 4-7-8 Breath: Health Benefits & Demonstration - DrWeil
..." 2012. <http://www.drweil.com/drw/u/VDR00112/The-4-7-8-
Breath-Benefits-and-Demonstration.html>

-"8 Reasons Why We Use Ujjayi Breath in Yoga." 2012.
<http://www.mindbodygreen.com/0-5823/8-Reasons-Why-We-
Use-Ujjayi-Breath-in-Yoga.html>

-"Nadi Shodhana – Channel Clearing Breath | The Chopra ..."
2014. <http://www.chopra.com/nadi-shodhana-channel-clearing-
breath>

-"Mindful Yoga Therapy for Veterans with Post Traumatic ..."
2011. <http://mindfulyogatherapy.org/>

-"Mindful"FOODMATTERS® | Find All You Need To Recharge
Your ..." 2008. 28 Jan. 2015 <http://www.foodmatters.tv/>ness
Meditation - Guided Mindfulness Meditation ..." 2004.
<http://www.mindfulnesscds.com/>

-"Health Journeys: Guided Meditation | Guided Imagery."
<http://www.healthjourneys.com/>

-"Marine Corps Studying How Mindfulness Meditation Can ..."
2013. <http://www.huffingtonpost.com/2013/01/22/marine-
corps-mindfulness-meditation_n_2526244.html>

-"Discover How to Use EFT Tapping, a Combination of ..." 2009.
<http://www.thetappingsolution.com/>

-"Tapping World Summit 2014." 2009.
<http://www.tappingworldsummit.com/>

-"Young Living | World Leader in Essential Oils."
<http://www.youngliving.com/>

-"dōTERRA - Essential Oils." 2006. 23 Jan. 2015
<http://www.doterra.com/>

-"Bonnie Blue Rescue." 2008. 7 Feb. 2015
<http://bonniebluerescue.com/>

-"Pet adoption: Want a dog or cat? Adopt a pet on Petfinder."
2009. <https://www.petfinder.com/>

-"Anti-Inflammatory Diet - Dr. Weil." 2007.
<http://www.drweil.com/drw/u/ART02012/anti-inflammatory-
diet>

-"Kris Carr, New York Times best-selling author and wellness."
<http://kriscarr.com/>

-"FOODMATTERS® | Find All You Need To Recharge Your ..."
2008. <http://www.foodmatters.tv/>

-"Wellness Mama | Simple Answers for Healthier Families."
2007. <http://wellnessmama.com/>

-"Greenspring Colonhydrotherapy - Home - Owings Mills, MD."
2009 <http://www.greenspringcolonhydrotherapy.com/>

-"Probiotics Benefits, Foods and Supplements - DrAxe.com."
2014. <http://draxe.com/probiotics-benefits-foods-
supplements/>

-"Kefir." 7 Feb. 2015 <http://www.kefir.net/>

-"Probiotic Drinks | KeVita Sparkling, Organic, Vegan
Beverages." 2008. <http://kevita.com/>

-"25 Surprising Ways Stress Affects Your Health - Health.com."
2012.
<http://www.health.com/health/gallery/0,,20642595,00.html>

-"Recover from Adrenal Burnout and Boost Your Energy."
2014. <http://www.integrativehealthcare.com/increase-energy/>

-"IAN WASTI | Creating Perspective." 2014.
<http://www.ianwasti.com/>

Chapter 4: Flexibility for Warriors

-"ACE-sponsored Study: Hot Yoga—Go Ahead and Turn Up."
2013. <https://www.acefitness.org/prosourcearticle/3353/ace-
sponsored-study-hot-yoga-go-ahead-and>
-"Ki-Hara Resistance Stretching - Innovative Body Solutions."
2008. <http://ki-hara.com/>
-"New Runner: Dynamic Stretching vs. Static Stretching." 2014.
<http://running.competitor.com/2014/07/injury-
prevention/dynamic-stretching-vs-static-stretching_54248>
-"Stretch Out Straps | Shop OPTP.com." 2013.
<http://www.optp.com/Stretch-Out-Straps>
-"Take a Trip to the SPA with YogaFit's Seven Principles of ..."
2013. <http://www.yogafit.com/news/blog/take-a-trip-to-the-
spa-with-yogafit-s-seven-principles-of-alignment/>
-"YogaFit - Yoga Teacher Training & Yoga Instructor ..."
<http://www.yogafit.com/>
-"The Stick." 2006. <https://www.thestick.com/>
-"Self Massage Therapy Balls - Yoga Tune Up." 2013.
<https://www.yogatuneup.com/self-massage-therapy-balls-
programs>
-"Yoga Tune Up®." 2010. 27 <https://www.yogatuneup.com/>
-"The NEW Art of Self-Care | MELT Method | Natural Pain
Relief." 2006. <http://www.meltmethod.com/>
-"MobilityWOD | All human beings should be able to perform
..." 2010. <http://www.mobilitywod.com/>
-"Trigger Point Performance Therapy." 2012.
<https://www.tptherapy.com/>
-"RumbleRoller Home." 2009.
<http://www.rumbleroller.com/>
-"Search Results | Shop OPTP.com." <http://www.optp.com/>
-"What is ChiRunning? - Chi Running." 2011.
<http://www.chirunning.com/what-is-chirunning/>

Chapter 5: Eat for Flexibility

-"Bio-individuality - Institute for Integrative Nutrition." 2014. <http://www.integrativenutrition.com/blog/2013/03/notes-from-iin%E2%80%99s-founder-why-it%E2%80%99s-ok-to-quit-being-vegan-or-macrobiotic>

-"Nourishing Wisdom." 2003. <http://nourishingwisdom.com/>

-"Crowding Out - Institute for Integrative Nutrition." 2014.

-"The Flexitarian Diet - Dawn Jackson Blatner, RD." 2011. <http://dawnjacksonblatner.com/books/the-flexitarian-diet/>

-"The Omnivore's Dilemma | Michael Pollan." 2010. <http://michaelpollan.com/books/the-omnivores-dilemma/>

-"DrWeil.com - Official Website of Andrew Weil, M.D." <http://www.drweil.com/>

-"Anti-Inflammatory Diet & Pyramid - DrWeil.com." 2008. <http://www.drweil.com/drw/u/PAG00361/anti-inflammatory-food-pyramid.html>

-"Natural Vibrant Health: Welcome." 2009. 3 Feb. 2015 <http://www.naturalvibranthealth.net/>

-"FOODMATTERS® | Find All You Need To Recharge Your ..." 2008. <http://www.foodmatters.tv/>

-"Kris Carr, New York Times best-selling author and wellness ..." 2005. <http://kriscarr.com/>

-"David Wolfe." <http://www.davidwolfe.com/>

-"How much omega-3 is enough? That depends on omega-6." 2011. <http://chriskresser.com/how-much-omega-3-is-enough-that-depends-on-omega-6>

-"HOOKED ON HEALTH - Empowering you to live a happier ..." 2014. <http://www.hookedonhealth.co/>

-"Welcome to the Blood Type Diet." <http://www.dadamo.com/>

-"Robb Wolf." 2007. <http://robbwolf.com/>

-"Chris Kresser – Let's take back your health - Starting Now." 2005. <http://chriskresser.com/>

-"Your Thyroid Pharmacist - Home | Hashimoto's ..." 2013. <http://www.thyroidpharmacist.com/>

-"Thyroid - Amy Myers MD." 2015.
<http://www.amymyersmd.com/2013/02/10-signs-you-have-a-thyroid-problem-and-10-solutions-for-it/>

-"Does Red Meat Cause Inflammation? - Chris Kresser." 2013.
<http://chriskresser.com/does-red-meat-cause-inflammation>

-"Why Go Vegetarian or Vegan? | Vegetarian Times." 2012.
<http://www.vegetariantimes.com/article/why-go-veg-learn-about-becoming-a-vegetarian/>

-"Taming Inflammation | How to Tame Inflammation ..." 2012.
<http://www.vegetariantimes.com/article/ask-the-doc-fire-starters/>

-"The Rich Roll Podcast #016: James 'Lightning' Wilks | Rich ..."
2013. <http://www.richroll.com/podcast/16-james-lightning-wilks/>

-"No Meat Athlete: Run on Plants and Discover Your Fittest ..."
2013. <http://www.nomeatathlete.com/book-info/>

-"Venus Williams uses plant-based vegan diet to combat ..."
2013. <http://www.examiner.com/article/venus-williams-talks-sjogren-s-syndrome-vegan-diet-with-dr-oz>

-"official site of Brendan Brazier." 2002.
<http://www.brendanbrazier.com/>

-"Home - Ben Greenfield Fitness - Fat Loss, Performance And
..." 2008. <http://www.bengreenfieldfitness.com/>

-"POWERED BY GREEN SMOOTHIES." 2010. 5 Feb. 2015
<http://poweredbygreensmoothies.com/>

-"How To Eat Organic On A Budget - Food Babe." 2013.
<http://foodbabe.com/2013/05/20/how-to-eat-organic-on-a-budget/>

-"Acidifying Foods & Inflammation | LIVESTRONG.COM." 2011.
<http://www.livestrong.com/article/548288-acidifying-foods-inflammation/>

-"4 Steps to Reducing Chronic Inflammation | Martha Stewart."
2011. <http://www.wholeliving.com/134407/4-steps-reducing-chronic-inflammation>

-"Nine Strategies to Reduce Inflammation - Rodale News."
2013. 16 Jan. 2015 <http://www.rodalenews.com/reduce-inflammation>

-"Dr. Mark Hyman: Home." 2005. 5 Feb. 2015
<http://drhyman.com/>

-"The Immune System Recovery Plan | Blum Center for
Health." 2014. 5 Feb. 2015 <http://blumcenterforhealth.com/the-
immune-system-recovery-plan/>

-"Amy Myers MD." 2013. 5 Feb. 2015
<http://www.amymyersmd.com/>

-"DrAxe.com: Home." 2005. 5 Feb. 2015 <http://draxe.com/>

-"Lissa Rankin |." 2005. 5 Feb. 2015 <http://lissarankin.com/>

-"Elimination Diet and Food Challenge Test for Diagnosing ..."
2012. 13 Feb. 2015
<http://www.webmd.com/allergies/guide/allergies-elimination-
diet>

-"JERF: Just Eat Real Food! | Underground Wellness." 2011. 6
Feb. 2015 <http://undergroundwellness.com/just-eat-real-food/>

-"Factory Farmed vs Wild Salmon | Mark's Daily Apple." 2008.
5 Feb. 2015 <http://www.marksdailyapple.com/salmon-factory-
farm-vs-wild/>

-"The Differences Between Grass-Fed Beef and Grain-Fed ..."
2011. 5 Feb. 2015 <http://www.marksdailyapple.com/the-
differences-between-grass-fed-beef-and-grain-fed-beef/>

-"Comparing Vitamin, Mineral and Energy Content of GMO vs
..." 2013. 5 Feb. 2015
<http://preventdisease.com/news/13/041613_Comparing-GMO-
to-Non-GMO-Vitamins-Minerals-Energy.shtml>

-"Oak Spring Farm." 2012. 11 Feb. 2015 <http://oakspring-
farm.com/>

-"Eggs Not Always What They're Cracked Up to Be ..." 2014. 11
Feb. 2015 <http://www.cornucopia.org/2014/12/eggs-not-
always-theyre-cracked/>

-"10 Proven Health Benefits of Eggs - Authority Nutrition."
2014. 11 Feb. 2015 <http://authoritynutrition.com/10-proven-
health-benefits-of-eggs/>

-"Dirty Dozen - Environmental Working Group." 2013. 5 Feb.
2015 <http://www.ewg.org/foodnews/summary.php>

-"The Simple Elimination Diet That Could Change Your Life ..."
2014. 6 Feb. 2015 <http://www.mindbodygreen.com/0-

12540/the-simple-elimination-diet-that-could-change-your-life-forever.html>

-"How too much omega-6 and not enough omega-3 is making ..." 2011. 15 Feb. 2015 <http://chriskresser.com/how-too-much-omega-6-and-not-enough-omega-3-is-making-us-sick>

-"Dr. Hyman's Discussion about Omega-3 Fats on the Dr. Oz ..." 2012. 6 Feb. 2015 <http://drhyman.com/blog/2011/01/18/dr-oz-show-omega-3-fats/>

-"Maroon, JC. "Omega-3 fatty acids (fish oil) as an anti-inflammatory: an ..." 2006. <http://www.ncbi.nlm.nih.gov/pubmed/16531187>

-"5 Superfoods that Fight Inflammation - Dr. Frank Lipman." 2013. 6 Feb. 2015 <http://www.drfranklipman.com/5-superfoods-that-fight-inflammation/>

-"Superfood Expert David Wolfe Shares Latest Insights on ..." 2010. 14 Jan. 2015 <http://articles.mercola.com/sites/articles/archive/2010/07/17/superfood-expert-david-wolfe-shares-latest-insights-on-how-to-stay-healthy.aspx>

-"Bone Broth: One of Your Most Healing Diet Staples - Mercola." 2013. 6 Feb. 2015 <http://articles.mercola.com/sites/articles/archive/2013/12/16/bone-broth-benefits.aspx>

-"Julie Daniluk | Meals That Heal Inflammation | Books | Julie ..." 2013. 6 Feb. 2015 <https://juliedaniluk.com/books/meals-that-heal-inflammation-by-julie-daniluk.html>

-"The Autoimmune Paleo Cookbook." 2013. 12 Feb. 2015 <http://autoimmune-paleo.com/cookbook/>

-"All Set for Surgery? - DrWeil.com." 2006. 6 Feb. 2015 <http://www.drweil.com/drw/u/id/QAA400056>

-"10 Superfoods You Should Be Eating - Simple Green ..." 2013. 10 Feb. 2015 <http://simplegreensmoothies.com/green-smoothie-superfoods>

-"Semper Fidelis Health and Wellness | Veteran Assistance ..." 2010. 9 Feb. 2015 <http://www.semperfidelishealthandwellness.org/>

-"Green Tea Health Benefits - WebMD." 2009. 6 Feb. 2015 <http://www.webmd.com/food-recipes/features/health-benefits-of-green-tea>

-"101 Uses for Coconut Oil - Wellness Mama." 2012. 6 Feb. 2015 <http://wellnessmama.com/5734/101-uses-for-coconut-oil/>

-"Sunwarrior: The Best Vegan Protein Powders and Plant ..." 2005. 9 Feb. 2015 <http://www.sunwarrior.com/>

-"Navitas Naturals - The Superfood Company ..." 2004. 9 Feb. 2015 <http://navitasnaturals.com/>

-"Dr. Oz's Favorite Tea Recipes | The Dr. Oz Show." 2014. 6 Feb. 2015 <http://www.doctoroz.com/recipe-collection/dr-ozs-favorite-tea-recipes>

-"11 Health Benefits of Dandelion and Dandelion Root ..." 2013. 10 Feb. 2015 <http://www.sunwarrior.com/news/11-health-benefits-of-dandelion-and-dandelion-root/>

-"Sunwarrior: The Best Vegan Protein Powders and Plant ..." 2005. 23 Feb. 2015 <http://www.sunwarrior.com/>

-"Dr. William Davis | Cardiologist & Author of Wheat Belly Books." 2011. 14 Feb. 2015 <http://www.wheatbellyblog.com/>

-"Gluten-Free can be Bad for 99% of Us. | elephant journal." 2013. 6 Feb. 2015 <http://www.elephantjournal.com/2013/05/gluten-free-can-be-bad-for-99-of-us/>

-"Anti-Inflammatory Herbs - Dr. Andrew Weil." 2009. 14 Jan. 2015 <http://www.drweil.com/drw/u/QAA142972/Anti-Inflammatory-Herbs.com>

-"Superfood Expert David Wolfe Shares Latest Insights on ..." 2010. 14 Jan. 2015 <http://articles.mercola.com/sites/articles/archive/2010/07/17/superfood-expert-david-wolfe-shares-latest-insights-on-how-to-stay-healthy.aspx>

-"Dr Carolyn Dean MD ND." 2007. 6 Feb. 2015 <http://drcarolyndean.com/>

-"Top 10 Magnesium Rich Foods Plus Proven Benefits - Dr. Axe." 2014. 6 Feb. 2015 <http://draxe.com/magnesium-deficient-top-10-magnesium-rich-foods-must-eating/>

-"Multivitamins and Supplements May Contain Toxic Selenite."
2011. 6 Feb. 2015
<http://articles.mercola.com/sites/articles/archive/2011/08/22/
is-your-multivitamin-toxic.aspx>
-"Adaptogens: Nature's Miracle Anti-stress and Fatigue
Fighters." 2012. 15 Jan. 2015
<http://www.drfranklipman.com/adaptogens-natures-miracle-
anti-stress-and-fatigue-fighters/>
-"Inflammatory Foods: 9 Of The Worst Picks For
Inflammation." 2013. 6 Feb. 2015
<http://www.huffingtonpost.com/2013/03/21/inflammatory-
foods-worst-inflammation_n_2838643.html>
-Wang, JJ. "Effects of moderate alcohol consumption on
inflammatory ..." 2008.
http://www.ncbi.nlm.nih.gov/pubmed/18372583

Additional Credits:

-"Bio-individuality" and "Crowding out" are trademarks that
are owned by Integrative Nutrition Inc.
www.integrativenutrition.com
-The "Dirty Dozen and Clean 15" list are trademarks of The
Environmental Working Group, a non-profit, non-partisan
organization dedicated to protecting human health and the
environment. EWG helps protect your family from pesticides!
Donate $10 at www.ewg.org and get the Shopper's Guide to
Pesticides in Produce™

Flexible Warrior Resources

Books:

Crazy Sexy Diet: Eat Your Veggies, Ignite Your Spark and Live Like You Mean It! by Kris Carr

Hashimoto's Thyroiditis: Lifestyle Interventions for Finding and Treating the Root Cause by Izabella Wentz, PharmaD, FASCP

Meals That Heal Inflammation: Embrace Healthy Living and Eliminate Pain, One Meal at a Time by Julie Daniluk

Nourishing Wisdom: A Mind-Body Approach to Nutrition and Well-Being by Marc David

One Word That Will Change Your Life by Jon Gordon, Dan Britton and Jimmy Page

Superfoods: The Food and Medicine Of The Future by David Wolfe

The Autoimmune Paleo Cookbook: An Allergen-Free Approach to Managing Chronic Illness by Mickey Trescott

The Athlete's Guide To Yoga: An Integrated Approach To Strength, Flexibility & Focus by Sage Rountree

The Flexitarian Diet: The Mostly Vegetarian Way to Lose Weight, Be Healthier, Prevent Disease and Add Years to Your Life by Dawn Blattner Jackson

The Magnesium Miracle by Dr. Carolyn Dean

The Omnivore's Dilema: A Natural History of Four Meals by Michael Pollen

8 Weeks To Optimum Health: A Proven Program for Taking Full Advantage of Your Body's Natural Healing Power by Dr. Andrew Weil

Wherever You Go There You Are: Mindfulness Meditation in Everyday Life by Jon Kabat Zinn

YogaLean: Poses and Recipes to Promote Weight Loss and Vitality for Life by Beth Shaw

Farmers Markets, CSA & Environment:

Local Harvest: www.localharvest.org

Farmers Market: www.farmersmarketonline.com

Environmental Working Group: www.ewg.org

Web Sites / Movies:

FOODMATTERS: www.foodmatters.tv

Hunger For Change: www.hungerforchange.tv

Food, Inc.: www.takepart.com

The Food Revolution Network: www.foodrevolution.org

Powered by Green Smoothies: www.poweredbygreensmoothies.com

Paleo / Primal Diet Experts:

Robb Wolf: www.robbwolf.com

Chris Kesser: www.chriskesser.com

Mark Sisson: www.marksdailyapple.com

Anti-inflammatory Diet:

Dr. Andrew Weil: www.drweil.com

Dr. Josh Axe www.draxe.com

Flexitarian Diet:

Dawn Jackson Blatner: www.dawnjacksonblatner.com

Raw / Vegan Athletes:

Brendan Brazier: www.brendanbrazier.com

Rich Roll: www.richroll.com

Matt Frazier: www.nomeatathlete.com

Venus Williams: www.venuswilliams.com

Raw Food, Superfoods, Superherbs & Supplements:

David Wolfe: www.davidwolfe.com

Kris Carr: www.kriscarr.com

Kendell Reichhart: www.naturalvibranthealth.com

Dr. Brian Clement: www.hippocratesinst.org

Non-Profit Organizations:

Warrior Wellness Services
www.semperfidelishealthandwellness.org

Believe Big www.believebig.org

Knights of Heroes www.knightsofheroes.org

Back On My Feet www.backonmyfeet.org

Podcasts & Online Resources:

Wellness Mama: www.wellnessmama.com

Tapping World Summit: www.tappingworldsummit.com

Sean Croxton/Underground Wellness:
www.undergroundwellness.com

Ben Greenfield Fitness: www.bengreenfieldfitness.com

Self-Care:

Essential Oils:

       Young Living: www.youngliving.com

       dōTERRA Essential Oils: www.doterra.com

Bio-Mat: www.therichwayBio-Mat.com

Guided Meditations by Belleruth Naperstack: www.healthjourneys.com

Colon Hydrotherapy: International Association of Colon Therapists: www.i-act.org

Yoga and Body Workers:

Yoga Teachers: www.yogaalliance.org

Massage Therapists: www.amtamassage.org

Acupuncture: www.medicalacupunture.org

Chiropractic: www.chiropractic.org

Rescue Animals:

Bonnie Blue Rescue: www.bonniebluerescue.com

Petfinder: www.petfinder.com

ASPCA: www.aspca.org

Humane Society: www.humanesociety.org

<u>Trainings:</u>

ACE Fitness: www.acefitness.org

Yogafit: www.yogafit.com

Spinning: www.spinning.com

Integrative Institute of Nutrition:
www.integrativenutrition.com

Ki-Hara: www.ki-hara.com

Intrinsic Health Systems: www.intrinsichealthsystems.com

<u>Self-Myofascial Release and Flexibility Products/Resources:</u>

Flexible Warrior Foam Roll & Stretch DVD:
www.spinervals.com

Stretch Out Strap: www.optp.com

RumbleRoller: www.rumberoller.com

TriggerPoint Performance Therapy: www.tptherapy.com

The Stick: www.thestick.com

Yoga Tune Up Therapy Balls: www.yogatuneup.com

Foam Rollers: www.performbetter.com

MobilityWOD: www.mobilitywod.com

The MELT Method: www.meltmethod.com

Functional Medicine / Alternative Doctors:

Dr. Wayne Bonlie: www.waynebonliemd.com

Dr. Mark Hyman: www.drhyman.com

Dr. Susan Blum: www.blumcenterforhealth.com

Dr. Amy Myers: www.amymyersmd.com

Dr. Josh Axe: www.draxe.com

Dr. Lissa Rankin: www.lissarankin.com

Dr. Joseph Mercola: www.mercola.com

Dr. Izabella Wentz: www.thyroidpharmacist.com

Suzy Cohen, RPh: www.suzycohen.com

Dr. Carolyn Dean: www.drcarolyndean.com

Functional Medicine Directory: www.functionalmedicine.org

The American Association of Drugless Practitioners: www.aadp.net

About the Author

Karen Dubs is a registered yoga teacher, a certified Pilates and Spinning instructor, a personal stretcher and a health coach specializing in flexibility, balance and recovery. She produced the Flexible Warrior Athletic Yoga DVD series with Spinervals and has taught yoga and stretching multiple seasons for The Baltimore Ravens football team and the University of Maryland Terrapins men's basketball team, in addition to private and group sessions for runners, triathletes, golfers, lacrosse and soccer players. Karen helped Olympic Pentathlete Suzanne Stettinius stay recovered and flexible while training for five sports leading up to the 2012 London Olympic games.

Karen enjoys teaching fundraiser yoga classes for her favorite charity organizations, Believe Big, Knights of Heroes and Back On My Feet. She also loves teaching Flexibility for Warriors sessions at Charm City Run in Baltimore and doing private recovery, stretch and mash sessions with athletes of all levels and sports.

Karen is a 1992 graduate of Towson University, where she majored in Mass Communications. She was born and raised in Hanover, Pennsylvania and lives near Baltimore, Maryland with her husband, Jon, and their rescue pup Stella.

The Flexible Warrior Athletic Yoga DVD series is available at www.spinervals.com

Free video segments at:
www.youtube.com/flexiblewarrioryoga

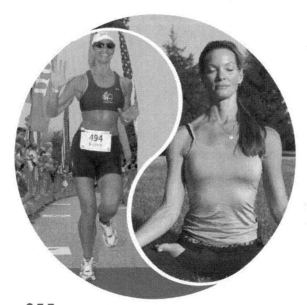

willpower
chillpower

Made in the USA
Charleston, SC
15 April 2015